Aids to Pathology

Dr. — Abood

Aids to Pathology

Michael F. Dixon

MB ChB MRC Path
Formerly SHO/Registrar in Pathology,
Royal Infirmary, Edinburgh; Formerly
Lecturer in Pathology, University
of Edinburgh; Lecturer in Pathology,
University of Leeds.

CHURCHILL LIVINGSTONE
EDINBURGH LONDON AND NEW YORK 1978

CHURCHILL LIVINGSTONE
Medical Division of Longman Group Limited

Distributed in the United States of America by
Longman Inc., 19 West 44th Street, New York,
N.Y. 10036 and by associated companies,
branches and representatives throughout
the world.

First published 1978

ISBN 0 443 014655

British Library Cataloguing in Publication Data.

Dixon, Michael F
　Aids to pathology.
　1. Pathology .
　I. Title
　616.07　　　　RB111　　　　77–30519

Printed in Singapore by
Kyodo-Shing Loong Printing Industries Pte. Ltd.

Preface

This book is intended as an easily assimilated revision guide to pathology. I have been motivated to write a book of this kind by a personal liking for listed information when preparing for examinations, and by the popularity of its companion volumes covering other medical specialities.

I have aimed at a comprehensive and, more importantly, comprehensible presentation of the major aspects of pathology. The text is a distillate of numerous books and articles and I claim no originality for most of the material which it contains. I have endeavoured, however, to arrange this material in a consistent and logical manner in the hope that the concentrated product will be more readily absorbed.

General pathology is covered in sufficient detail to meet the requirements of any undergraduate examination and the primary examinations of the Royal Colleges. Systemic pathology receives more concise treatment but conditions of major clinical importance, or those popular with examiners, are dealt with in greater detail. Fuller accounts of all the topics covered, including relevant clinical and experimental information, can be found in the books cited as General References. For those students seeking greater detail, and in particular postgraduates taking higher qualifications in pathology, I have listed helpful review articles, monographs and specialised text-books, at the end of chapters.

It is a pleasure to acknowledge the help of my colleagues in the Department of Pathology, in particular Dr A.J. Franks and Dr R.W. Blewitt, who made many useful comments on the manuscript. I am also grateful to Mrs K. Hewitt for secretarial assistance, and to my publisher at Churchill Livingstone for his helpful advice.

1978   M.F.D.

Contents

The cell and cell injury 1

Acute inflammation 12

Healing 22

Chronic inflammation 29

Immunopathology 36

Resistance to infection 47

Granulomatous diseases 52

Hypertension 66

Atherosclerosis and aneurysms 74

Thrombosis and embolism 79

Oedema and congestion 88

The effects of injury on the body 93

Congenital malformations 96

Inborn errors of metabolism 99

Disorders of body pigments 105

Calcification 113

Amyloid 115

Atrophy, hypertrophy and hyperplasia 120

Metaplasia, dysplasia and carcinoma-in-situ 124

Neoplasia 128

Biological effects of radiation 143

Alimentary system 146

Liver, gall-bladder and pancreas 162

Cardiovascular system 173

Respiratory system 181

Genito-urinary system 193

Lymphoid tissue 209

Endocrine system 212

Musculoskeletal system 222

Auto-immune diseases 230

Nervous system 233

General references 242

Index 243

The cell and cell injury

STRUCTURE AND FUNCTION OF CELL COMPONENTS

Nucleus

The nucleus is composed principally of deoxyribonucleic acid (DNA) in combination with a protein (histone) within a ground substance. The nucleic acid material (chromatin) stains well with basic dyes such as haematoxylin and methylene blue, and DNA can be stained specifically by the Feulgen technique. Chromatin patterns vary from cell to cell. The plasma cell, for example, has a distinctive 'cartwheel' pattern. The nucleus is separated from the cytoplasm by a double membrane—*the nuclear envelope*—containing circular holes 50 to 70 nm in diameter—*nuclear pores*.

The pores, which are usually crossed by a diffuse membrane, probably represent the sites of interchange between nucleus and cytoplasm.

Functions of the nucleus
1. Replication of DNA
2. Production of messenger RNA
3. Synthesis of some nuclear proteins

Nucleolus

The nucleus normally contains one or more small basophilic structures—nucleoli, composed of a dense network (nucleolonema) enclosing paler areas (the pars amorpha). The granules of the nucleolonema are thought to represent newly-synthesised ribosome subunits which pass out of the nucleus along with messenger RNA and direct the synthesis of specific proteins in the cytoplasm.

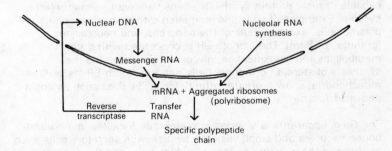

Cytoplasm

Cytosol differs from extracellular fluid in having a high concentration of potassium, magnesium and phosphate. Sodium is actively excluded by the ATP-dependent 'sodium-pump' across the cell membrane. Many functions reside in the cytosol or cytoplasmic matrix, namely:

1

1. Glycolysis
2. Some reactions in gluconeogenesis
3. Activation and synthesis of some amino acids
4. Fatty acid synthesis
5. Mononucleotide synthesis
6. Phosphogluconate pathway

Mitochondria

These round, ovoid, or sinuous cytoplasmic organelles possess a complete outer trilaminar membrane and an inner membrane which shows numerous infoldings termed cristae. Although all mitochondria have this basic structure there is considerable variability both in the number and length of the cristae and in the number and general outline of the mitochondria. Cells with a high metabolic activity have large mitochondria with numerous cristae, for example cardiac muscle and gastric parietal cells. In the liver, whilst the mitochondria are large, the cristae are sparse and irregular.

Mitochondria contain most of the enzymes of the citric acid cycle and the energy derived from the oxidation of acetylco-A in the cycle is used to convert adenosine diphosphate to triphosphate—oxidative phosphorylation.

Endoplasmic reticulum

All cells contain a system of complex paired membranes enclosing small vesicles or channels—the cisternae. These membranes form the endoplasmic reticulum (ER) and are either studded with ribosomes forming so-called rough ER or are devoid of granules and are termed smooth ER. The main function of the rough ER, together with free ribosomes in the cytoplasm, is protein synthesis. Protein produced by the rough ER is usually for export via the Golgi apparatus. Ribosomes are basophilic so that the cytoplasm of cells capable of rapid protein synthesis stains well with haematoxylin or pyronin. Examples of cells showing such cytoplasmic basophilia are plasma cells, exocrine cells of the pancreas, and hepatocytes (granules of Berg). The smooth ER is concerned with drug metabolism and detoxification, glycogen synthesis, and the synthesis of steroid hormones. Cells rich in smooth ER (as well as mitochondria) show a greater affinity for acidic dyes such as eosin and acid fuchsin.

The Golgi apparatus is a series of membrane lamellae, membrane-bound vacuoles and small vesicles, best seen in secretory cells such as those of the exocrine pancreas, goblet cells, and the absorptive cells of the gut. The Golgi is thought to package secretions which reach it through the cisternae of the ER. The secretion granules then bud off and migrate to the apex of the cell.

Lysosomes are rounded, membrane-bound bodies showing wide variation in their size, shape, and internal structure. They are the main components of an intracellular digestive system and contain numerous hydrolases active at acid pH, such as phosphatase, betaglucuronidase, esterases, ribonuclease and deoxyribonuclease. The digestive activity is generally contained within the lysosomes themselves. In *heterophagy* exogenous material enters the cell by endocytosis and the vacuole thus formed fuses with primary lysosomes, probably produced by the Golgi apparatus. In *autophagy,* damaged cytoplasmic components are enveloped to form an autophagic vacuole which fuses with primary lysosomes. Digestion proceeds in the secondary lysosomes so-formed and products diffuse out to be re-utilised by the cell. Undigested material can in some instances be expelled by exocytosis, otherwise it remains in the cell as a residual dense body.

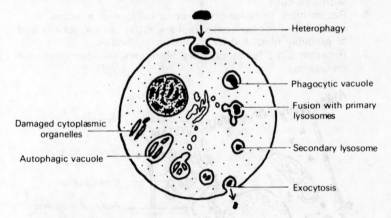

Lysosomes are important in:
1. Polymorphs and macrophages in killing and digesting infective agents
2. Protein reabsorption in the kidney
3. Removal of unwanted cells during embryonic development
4. Disposal of excess secretory products in glandular cells
5. Osteoclastic remodelling of bone by secreted enzymes
6. Supply of nutrients, e.g. in liver.

Microbodies or peroxisomes consist of a homogeneous matrix sometimes containing a central crystalline nucleus enclosed in a single membrane. They contain a number of enzymes, including amino-acid oxidases, urate oxidase and catalase, and are most numerous in liver and kidney cells. Their role in the cell economy is obscure.

Cell membrane

Cells are enclosed by trilaminar or unit membrane composed of a sandwich of lipoprotein molecules. In addition to maintaining the integrity of the cytoplasm, the cell membrane has a number of important functions:

1. Intake of exogenous material by phagocytosis, pinocytosis or micropinocytosis
2. Selective permeability
3. The ATP-associated sodium-pump which actively shifts sodium ions across the membrane out of the cytoplasm
4. Cell-to-cell contact and adhesion by means of junctional complexes—tight junction, intermediate junction, and desmosome
5. Contact inhibition—the mechanism whereby further proliferation and movement of cells is inhibited by contact with like cells
6. Recognition. The capacity to recognise foreign antigens and altered or effete host cells, resides at the cell membrane and is probably mediated by cytophilic antibodies
7. Receptor sites for stimulatory hormones or other chemical mediators.

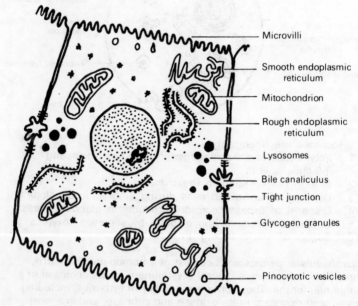

Microvilli

Smooth endoplasmic reticulum

Mitochondrion

Rough endoplasmic reticulum

Lysosomes

Bile canaliculus

Tight junction

Glycogen granules

Pinocytotic vesicles

Normal cell components: Hepatocyte

CAUSES OF CELL INJURY

1. Toxic substances

    (i)   General—e.g. corrosives and phenol which denature protein

    (ii)   Tissue specific—e.g. carbon tetrachloride producing liver necrosis; alloxan giving rise to necrosis in ß cells of the pancreatic islets

    (iii) Biochemically specific—enzyme poisons such as cyanide on cytochrome oxidase; sodium fluoracetate block of the Krebs cycle

2. Physical agents

    (i)   Trauma

    (ii)   Heat

    (iii) Cold

    (iv) Ionising radiation

3. Lack of nutrients

Local

    (i)   Failure of cellular absorption, e.g. glucose in diabetes mellitus

    (ii)   Ischaemia

General

    (i)   Hypoxia, e.g. severe anaemia, respiratory failure

    (ii)   Dietary deficiency or malabsorption

    (iii) Hormonal deficiency

4. Infective agents and parasites

Injure by

    (i)   Production of toxins

    (ii)   Competition for essential nutrients

    (iii) Provocation of hypersensitivity reactions

    (iv) Intracellular multiplication

5. Immune mechanisms

    (i)   Auto-immune diseases

    (ii)   Hypersensitivity states, e.g. contact dermatitis

6. Genetic defects

    (i)   Change in chromosome make-up

         a. Alteration in number—aneuploidy

         b. Alteration in structure as a result of deletion or translocation

    (ii)   Change in genetic code leading for example to inborn errors of metabolism

EVOLUTION OF CELL INJURY

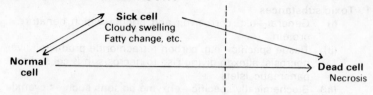

Injury to a cell may result in changes such as cloudy swelling and fat accumulation which, if the injurious agent is withdrawn, are reversible and the cell recovers. If, however, the injury persists the cell may degenerate further, become irreversibly damaged, and die. In some circumstances the injury may be so catastrophic that the cell dies without showing these intermediate changes.

When a noxious environment producing lesser degrees of cell injury persists, the cell may adapt to this altered environment and establish a new steady state. Only when the cell fails to establish an altered level of homeostasis in response to injury is cell death inevitable.

EFFECTS OF CELL INJURY

1. Injury to cell membranes and mitochondria

(i) Loss of microvilli and focal expansions of the plasma membrane

(ii) Disruption of the RER and loss of ribosomes. This brings about the loss of cytoplasmic basophilia seen on light microscopy

(iii) Mitochondrial swelling and loss of cristae

2. Cloudy swelling (intracellular oedema)

This results from the accumulation of watery fluid in the dilated sacs or cisternae of the endoplasmic reticulum and mitochondria.

(i) Early stages—under the light microscope the cytoplasm has a fine granularity like ground-glass

(ii) Later stages—progressive dilatation of the ER leads to the appearance of clear vacuoles visible by light microscopy—*hydropic vacuolation*

Mechanism

(i) Fall in oxidative phosphorylation due to
 a. Lack of oxygen
 b. Damage to mitochondria or its enzymatic pathways
The diminished formation of ATP affects all the energy requiring reactions in the cell but in particular leads to failure of the sodium-pump. Sodium ions enter the cell in exchange for potassium and as the former have a larger hydration shell, there is a net influx of water.

(ii) Increased intracellular osmotic pressure resulting from
 a. Accumulation of lactate and pyruvate
 b. Net catabolism of macromolecules

3. Fatty change

This is the appearance of abundant spherical globules of fat (triglyceride) within the cytoplasm. It can be demonstrated using frozen sections and staining with lipid-soluble dyes such as Oil red O or Sudan black, and is most commonly seen in cells of the liver, kidney and myocardium. Fatty change must be distinguished from pathological adiposity where fat cells (lipocytes) infiltrate an organ or tissue. This is a feature of severe obesity. In normal cells fat is held in a dispersed state and transported out of the cell as micelles or lipoprotein complexes (triglyceride with phospholipid and/or protein). Triglycerides are synthesised from free fatty acids (FFA's) entering the cell from the blood. FFA's also undergo oxidation to CO_2 and conversion to phospholipid.

Mechanism

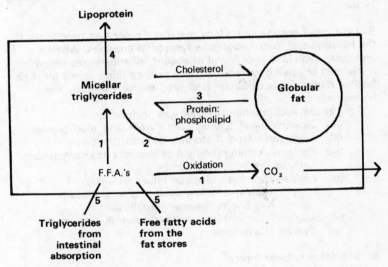

Fatty change results from:
- A. Impaired metabolism of fat
  - (i) Reduced oxidation of FFA's with increased conversion to triglycerides (**1**)
  - (ii) Reduced synthesis of phospholipid and protein (**2**). This results in
    - a. Reduced dispersal of fat (**3**)
    - b. Diminished release of fat from the cell as lipoprotein (**4**)
- B. Excessive entry of FFA's and triglyceride into the cell (**5**).

Causes

    (i)   Diabetes mellitus

    (ii) Congestive cardiac failure

    (iii) Severe anaemia

    (iv) Malnutrition and wasting disease

    (v) Ischaemia, e.g. coronary insufficiency

    (vi) Infections (septicaemia)

    (vii) Chronic alcoholism (liver)

    (viii) Poisons, e.g. carbon tetrachloride, phosphorus (liver)

4. Lysosomal damage

A. *Lysosomal rupture* is thought to be responsible for some forms of cell injury, e.g. injury to alveolar macrophages after phagocytosis of silica. In toxic injury, however, rupture is thought to be a consequence of advanced cellular damage rather than an initiating factor.

B. *Lysosomal overloading.* Many metabolic processes depend upon the hydrolysis of intermediates by lysosomal enzymes. When a particular hydrolase is deficient or absent, all substances entering lysosomes or arising within them that require this enzyme for their further digestion, accumulate and progressively enlarge the lysosome.

Substances accumulating in this way include:

    (i)   *Lipofuscin*—in ageing cells ('wear and tear' pigment)

    (ii) *Glycogen*—Type II storage disease (Pompe)

    (iii) *Protein*—forming the hyaline deposits in kidney tubule cells in the nephrotic syndrome

    (iv) *Lipids*—Gaucher's disease (glucoceramide)

            Niemann-Pick disease (sphingomyelin)

            Tay-Sachs disease (gangliosides)

    (v) *Mucopolysaccharide*—Hurler's syndrome (gargoylism)

    (vi) *Cystine*—cystinosis

5. Sublethal nuclear injury

Ionising radiation and certain chemical compounds such as the mustards and ethyleneimides exert their toxic effects principally on cell nuclei. High doses result in cell death, but smaller doses may produce:

    (i)   Mutations. Latent injury to DNA may result in mutation and the development of malignant cells.

    (ii) Genetic abnormalities. Similar injury to germ cells may produce changes in the DNA code which result in genetic abnormalities in the offspring.

CELL DEATH—NECROSIS

Features of the irreversible injury leading to cell death are:
1. Cessation of oxidative phosphorylation in the damaged mitochondria
2. Continued loss of potassium ions. Sodium and calcium ions enter the cell but eventually semi-permeability is lost and the accompanying influx of water ceases
3. Anaerobic glycolysis continues with a consequent fall in pH. This activates enzymes escaping from ruptured lysosomes and accelerates autolysis
4. Disordered metabolism of the cell leading to nuclear changes

Cell death is recognised by:
1. Changes in the nucleus
   (i) Swelling and clumping of chromatin
   (ii) Pyknosis—condensation of chromatin and shrinkage of the nucleus
   (iii) Karyorrhexis—fragmentation of the nucleus
   (iv) Karyolysis—dissolution of the nucleus by deoxyribonuclease
2. Changes in cytoplasmic staining
   (i) Positive staining with vital dyes such as trypan blue which reflects abnormal membrane permeability
   (ii) Opacification—denaturation of proteins leads to aggregation with resultant opacification of the cytoplasm
   (iii) Eosinophilia—exposure of basic amino groups results in increased affinity for acidic dyes such as eosin
3. Ultrastructural changes
   (i) Margination or progressive loss of nuclear chromatin
   (ii) Focal rupture of the nuclear membrane
   (iii) Breakdown of the plasmalemma
   (iv) Development of flocculent densities in mitochondria
4. Biochemical changes
   (i) Release of K^+ by dead cells
   (ii) Release of enzymes into the blood, e.g. increased plasma levels of creatine kinases, lactic dehydrogenase and aspartate aminotransferase (formerly GOT)
   (iii) Release of protein or protein breakdown products into the blood, e.g. myoglobin from injured skeletal muscle cells.

FORMS OF NECROSIS
A. General forms
1. Single cells
   (i) Apoptosis or shrinkage necrosis as in
       a. Cell death in physiological cell turnover
       b. Cell death in tumours
       c. Scattered cell death in certain infections, e.g. acidophil bodies in hepatitis
2. Multiple cells (tissues)
   (i) Coagulative necrosis
       a. Architecture preserved, e.g. renal infarct, syphilitic gumma
       b. Architecture destroyed, e.g. caseous necrosis in tuberculosis
   (ii) Colliquative necrosis—necrosis and liquefaction, e.g. cerebral infarct

B. Special forms
1. Gangrene
   (i) Dry gangrene—mummification, e.g. in a limb resulting from peripheral vascular disease
   (ii) Wet gangrene—necrosis and superadded infection e.g. in the small intestine following mesenteric thrombosis, gas-gangrene resulting from clostridial infection
2. Fat-necrosis
   (i) Traumatic—release of lipid from fat cells provokes a chronic inflammatory and giant cell response as seen in subcutaneous fat or in the breast
   (ii) Enzymatic—as occurs in association with acute pancreatitis
3. Fibrinoid 'necrosis'—this is not a true necrosis but a strongly eosinophilic degeneration of collagen, e.g. in a rheumatoid nodule; or in polyarteritis nodosa.

CONSEQUENCES OF NECROSIS
1. Acute inflammation
2. Healing by repair or regeneration
3. Chronic inflammation
4. Immunological reactions to subcellular components released by dead tissue, or to self-antigens altered by denaturation, e.g. the postmyocardial infarction syndrome
5. Calcification, e.g. in old caseous foci of tuberculosis

THE RELATIONSHIP OF CELL INJURY TO DISEASE

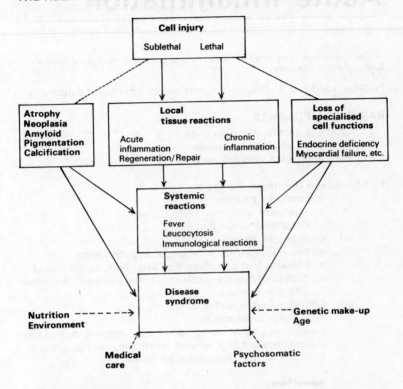

FURTHER READING

American Journal of Pathology (1975) The biochemical pathology of cell injury. Symposium in *American Journal of Pathology,* **81,** 162.

Dixon, K.C. (1970) Cell injury. In *A Companion to Medical Studies,* vol. 2, ed. Passmore, R. & Robson, J.S. Oxford: Blackwell.

Toner, P.G. & Carr, K.E. (1971) *Cell Structure,* 2nd edn. Edinburgh: Churchill Livingstone.

Acute inflammation

'A local response of living tissue to injury resulting in the formation of a protein-rich fluid and cellular exudate'.

Protein rich fluid + Phagocytic cells = 'Inflammatory exudate'

BASIC COMPONENTS
1. Changes in the microcirculation
2. Formation of a fluid exudate
3. Formation of a cellular exudate

1. Changes in the microcirculation
    (i)   Changes in calibre
        a. Transient arteriolar constriction
        b. Persistent vasodilatation
    (ii) Changes in flow
        a. Initially rapid as a result of vasodilatation
        b. Slowing and disturbance of axial flow as a result of increased blood viscosity secondary to loss of plasma into the tissue
    (iii) Changes in the endothelium
        a. Cellular contraction
        b. Becomes adhesive for leucocytes, possibly due to the development of a cement layer composed of either fibrin or acid mucopolysaccharide

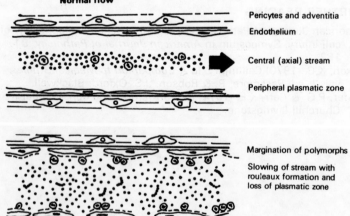

Normal flow

Pericytes and adventitia
Endothelium

Central (axial) stream

Peripheral plasmatic zone

Margination of polymorphs

Slowing of stream with rouleaux formation and loss of plasmatic zone

Acute inflammation

2. Formation of a fluid exudate

Normally the walls of small blood vessels are freely permeable to water and crystalloids but are relatively impermeable to plasma proteins. The formation of a protein-rich fluid exudate is facilitated by separation of the intercellular junctions of the endothelium. This change is maximal in small venules with a diameter of 20-30 μm. Having passed through the endothelium protein molecules can freely permeate the basement membrane, pericytes and adventitia.

The fluid exudate carries into the inflamed area the following important constituents:

- (i) Serum bactericidal factors
  - a. Antibodies which act by opsonising bacteria prior to phagocytosis and by neutralising exotoxins
  - b. Components of the complement system (see p. 14)
- (ii) Interferon: a non-specific antiviral agent
- (iii) Fibrinogen which is converted to fibrin
  Fibrin is important in providing
  - a. Cement substance uniting severed tissues
  - b. 'Scaffold' for repair processes
  - c. Barrier to the spread of organisms
  - d. Surface against which phagocytosis of adherent organisms is enhanced
- (iv) Therapeutic agents—antibiotics, anti-inflammatory drugs, etc.

Soon after the vascular changes of acute inflammation have commenced, leucocytes migrate through the walls of venules and veins and appear in the interstitium. Neutrophil polymorphs are the first to appear and take between 2 to 12 minutes to traverse the wall. They are followed by monocytes and small numbers of eosinophils.

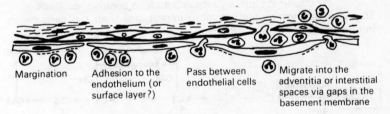

| Margination | Adhesion to the endothelium (or surface layer?) | Pass between endothelial cells | Migrate into the adventitia or interstitial spaces via gaps in the basement membrane |

Steps in polymorph emigration

3. Formation of the cellular exudate
The steps in leucocyte emigration are:
- (i) Appearance of polymorphs in the peripheral plasmatic zone in venules
- (ii) Margination or 'pavementing' of polymorphs along the endothelium
- (iii) Adhesion of polymorphs (and later, monocytes) to endothelial cells in the presence of divalent cations
- (iv) Leucocytes enlarge the gaps between endothelial cells and pass through by amoeboid motion
- (v) After a temporary hold-up the cells pass through gaps in the basement membrane where it divides to enclose pericytes

Leucocyte emigration is followed by a passive loss of red blood cells through the points of rupture, so-called *diapedesis*.

COMPLEMENT AND INFLAMMATION
1. The complement system
The system consists of 9 protein components (C1-C9) and a number of associated ions and co-factors. When the first component is activated by an immune complex (Ab-Ag) it initiates a sequence of pro-enzyme activation (C4, C2, C3, etc) in which there is considerable amplification at each step in the cascade. This is the 'classical' pathway.

The system can also be activated at the C3 level (the *alternate* pathway) by:
- (i) Activation of a proenzyme of C3 proactivator convertase by a variety of substances including endotoxin and aggregated IgA, IgE, and IgG_4
- (ii) C3b—a cleavage product of C3 generated by the classical pathway which acts as a positive feedback.

This pathway is probably of more importance than the classical in inflammation.

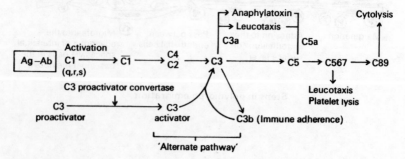

2. Activities of the complement system

Activation results in the production of a number of biologically active factors:

(i) Fragments (C3a and C5a) are released which augment the inflammatory response by causing histamine release (*anaphylatoxin*), and directing the migration of polymorphs (leucotaxis)

(ii) Complex C567 is chemotactic for polymorphs

(iii) Modified C3 molecules (C3b) opsonise particles and membranes permitting *immune adherence* with macrophages and platelets via their C3 receptor sites. This facilitates phagocytosis and may result in platelet aggregation

(iv) In addition to platelet aggregation by C3b, C567 complexes may bring about lysis of platelets and release of platelet factor XII. These actions may initiate blood coagulation.

(v) Activation of the terminal C8 and 9 produces cytolysis possibly through a phospholipase action on cell membranes

THE INFLAMMATORY MEDIATORS

A. Chemical agents increasing vascular permeability

1. *Amines*—Histamine, 5-hydroxytryptamine (5-HT)

(i) Storage—in granules of mast cells, basophils and platelets

(ii) Release provoked by:
   a. Anaphylaxis—IgE mediated
   b. Anaphylotoxins (C3a, C5a)
   c. Cytolysis by full complement sequence
   d. Prostaglandins

(iii) Action in the presence of calcium ions—rapid, but short-lived, important during the early phase of acute inflammation (30 – 90 min)

2. *Kinins*

(i) Nature—straight chained basic peptides of 9, 10, or 11 amino acids, e.g. bradykinin, kallidin

(ii) Formation—kinins are generated from an inactive plasma precursor kininogen by cleavage brought about by kallikrein. This in turn is generated by the action on kallikreinogen of plasmin or activated Factor XII Factor XII is activated by
   a. Surface contact
   b. Antigen – antibody complexes
   c. Bacterial endotoxin
   d. Permeability globulin (PF/dil)
   e. Polymorph lysosomal enzymes

(iii) Action—more prolonged than histamine, up to 2½ h.

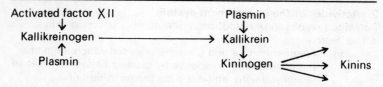

3. *Anaphylatoxins* (C3a, C5a)
   - (i)   Nature—arginine-rich peptides derived by cleavage of C3 and C5
   - (ii)   Action—potent, but short-lived as they are rapidly inactivated by a plasma carboxypeptidase. Cause release of histamine from mast cells
4. *Leucokinins*
   - (i)   Nature—peptides with molecular weights about 3600 derived from the action of a proteolytic enzyme from leucocytes (Leucokininogenase) on a plasma protein precursor
   - (ii)   Action—probably act by directly increasing vascular permeability
5. *Permeability globulin* (PF/dil)
   - (i)   Nature—a protein (possibly factor XII itself) which on dilution of plasma gives rise to a permeability factor
   - (ii)   Action—indirect effect mediated by activation of factor XII and subsequent production of kinins
6. *Slow-reacting substance of anaphylaxis* (SRS-A)
   - (i)   Nature—a small m.wt. substance (<2000) released following contact of sensitised tissues with antigen. Its production may be mediated by anaphylactic (IgE) antibodies
   - (ii)   Actions—increases vascular permeability and causes contraction of smooth muscle
7. *Prostaglandins*
   - (i)   Nature—a group of at least 13 long-chain fatty acids derived from a 20-carbon parent compound, prostanoic acid
   - (ii)   Action—prostaglandins E_1 and E_2 are thought to be important in sustaining the later phases of the inflammatory response and act in part by liberating histamine. There appears to be an inverse relationship between endogenous cyclic AMP (adenosine monophosphate) levels and the synthesis of prostaglandins

Summary
The early increase in vascular permeability (30 – 90 min) is brought about by *histamine* and *5-hydroxytryptamine*.

The intermediate phase (90 min—3 h) is mediated by plasma and leuco*kinins* and *anaphylatoxins.*

The later phase (3 h – 24 h+) is mediated by *SRS-A* and *prostaglandins.*

In some cases, increased capillary permeability results from direct injury to the endothelium.

B. Leucotactic factors

1. *Complement factors*
   - (i) Cleavage fragments of C3 and C5 similar to, but not identical with the anaphylatoxins C3a and C5a
   - (ii) The C567 complex is chemotactic for polymorphs

2. *Bacterial factors*
   - (i) Soluble low m.wt. products which are directly chemotactic
   - (ii) Bacterial proteases which cleave C3 and C5

3. *Tissue factors*
Tissue injury results in release of a C3 cleaving enzyme from the damaged cells

4. *Eosinophil chemotactic factor of anaphylaxis* (ECF-A)
A heat stable low m.wt substance released from sensitised mast-cells by exposure to antigen, for example in atopic reactions such as hay fever and urticaria.

ACTIVITIES OF THE NEUTROPHIL POLYMORPH

1. *Phagocytosis and bacterial killing*
   Stages:
   - (i) Chemotaxis
   - (ii) Adhesion usually following opsonisation, mainly by IgG, IgM and C3
   - (iii) Phagocytosis resulting in a membrane-bound vacuole enclosing the bacteria—the phagosome
   - (iv) Fusion of phagosome with lysosomes (granules)
   - (v) Bacterial killing by
     - a. Hydrogen peroxide (which is produced by the oxidation of glucose through the hexosemonophosphate shunt) in conjunction with halide ions (Cl^- or I^-), and myeloperoxidase
     - b. Granule lysozyme
     - c. Granule basic (cationic) proteins which attach themselves to the bacterial membrane
     - d. Lactic acid accumulation

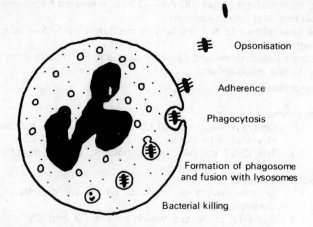

2. *Initiation of blood coagulation*
By release of lysosomal enzymes (degranulation) which activate factor XII.

3. *Tissue injury*
By release of lysosomal enzymes from dead and dying polymorphs.

4. *Release of pyrogens*
Which act on the hypothalamus and bring about a rise in body temperature.

DISORDERS OF POLYMORPHS

A. Defective production (neutropenia)
1. Drug-induced neutropenia
2. Associated with aplastic anaemia
3. Associated with acute leukaemia
4. Associated with splenomegaly
5. Immune neutropenia resulting from
   (i)   Multiple blood transfusions (anti-leucocyte antibodies)
   (ii) Passive maternal antibodies in neonates
   (iii) Auto-immune reactions in SLE, rheumatoid disease, etc.
6. Chronic infantile agranulocytosis
7. Chronic benign neutropenia of childhood
8. Associated with thymic aplasia or dysgammaglobulinaemia
9. Associated with exocrine pancreatic insufficiency (Schwachman's syndrome)

B. Defective chemotaxis
1.   Due to a cellular defect which in some cases may be related to increased cyclic AMP
     (i)   In neonates
     (ii)   Chediak-Higashi disease—an autosomal recessive condition characterised by partial albinism and recurrent bacterial infections
     (iii) In some patients with diabetes mellitus, rheumatoid arthritis and acute bacterial infections
     (iv)   In the mucocutaneous candidiasis syndrome
     (v)   Job's syndrome—children with eczema and recurrent 'cold' staphylococcal abscesses
2.   Due to a deficiency of the chemotactic factors derived from the complement system, i.e. C3 and C5 deficiency results in a lack of the active cleavage products
3.   Due to a chemotaxis inhibitor in the serum as has been found in Hodgkin's disease

C. Defective phagocytosis
1.   Defect in opsonization due to lack of complement, or to lack of IgM in neonate and hypogammaglobulinaemia
2.   Lack of non-specific stimulator of phagocytosis present in normal serum which acts on the neutrophil membrane ('tuftsin')

D. Defects in bactericidal activity
1.   Associated with established severe bacterial infection
2.   Chronic granulomatous disease of childhood due to defective H_2O_2 formation resulting in recurrent bacterial infections, granulomata in various sites and hepatosplenomegaly
3.   Chediak—Higashi disease—where in addition to the chemotactic defect the polymorphs contain giant lysosomes which fail to fuse with the phagosomes
4.   Myeloperoxidase deficiency
     (i)   Familial
     (ii)   Secondary to acute myeloid leukaemia
5.   Severe glucose-6-phosphate dehydrogenase deficiency in polymorphs
6.   Drug induced, e.g. corticosteroids
7.   In fulminant hepatic failure due to a serum inhibitor of the hexose monophosphate shunt

VARIETIES OF ACUTE INFLAMMATION

The general response to injury is modified according to the tissue and the nature of the injurious agent resulting in several descriptive types of inflammation.

1. *Serous*: formation of a protein-rich fluid exudate with minor cellular exudation, e.g. synovitis, peritonitis.

2. *Fibrinous*: exudate contains abundant fibrinogen which is precipitated as a thick fibrin coating, e.g. pericarditis.

3. *Haemorrhagic*: inflammation associated with conspicuous haemorrhage as a result of vascular damage, e.g. meningococcaemia, viral pneumonia.

4. *Suppurative* (or purulent)—characterised by the production of pus composed of:
    (i)   Dead and dying polymorphs
    (ii) Liquefied tissue
    (iii) Pyogenic organisms
Suppuration may result in the formation of:
    (i)   Abscess—a localised collection of pus in an organ or tissue
    (ii) Empyema—a collection of pus in a hollow viscus, e.g. in the gall-bladder or appendix

5. *Membranous*: inflammation of a lining epithelium with a coating of fibrinous exudate, more or less intact desquamated epithelium, and inflammatory cells.

6. *Pseudo-membranous*: the adherent coat is composed of matted fibrin and inflammatory cells and is usually associated with only focal superficial ulceration, e.g. pseudomembranous colitis due to clindamycin toxicity, or ischaemic injury.

7. *Catarrhal*: inflammation of mucosal surfaces with hypersecretion of mucus, e.g. common cold.

8. *Necrotising* (gangrenous): acute inflammation associated with widespread necrosis of the organ probably resulting from superimposed thrombosis or vascular occlusion due to high tissue pressure, e.g. in severe acute appendicitis.

OUTCOME OF ACUTE INFLAMMATION

1. *Resolution.* The inflammatory exudate is reabsorbed and the tissue restored to normal, e.g. lobar pneumonia. This presumes that there has been no tissue destruction.

2. *Healing* by repair or regeneration where tissue has been destroyed.

3. *Chronic inflammation*

4. *Spread*
    (i)   Direct—e.g. cellulitis
    (ii) Lymphatic—lymphangitis progressing to acute lymphadenitis
    (iii) Blood vessels
        a. Pyaemia—spread of pyogenic organisms in infected micro-thrombi via the blood stream possibly giving rise to secondary (metastatic) abscesses
        b. Septicaemia—multiplication of organisms in the blood stream in the absence of adequate host defences

5. *Death* resulting from
    (i) Toxaemia, e.g. endotoxic shock and its complications
    (ii) Involvement of vital organs, e.g. encephalitis, myocarditis

FURTHER READING

Hurley, J.V. (1972) *Acute Inflammation.* Edinburgh: Churchill Livingstone.
Ryan, G.B. & Majno, G. (1977) Acute inflammation. *American Journal of Pathology,* **86,** 183.

Healing

Healing is the replacement of destroyed or lost tissue by viable tissue. It is achieved in two ways:
1. *Repair.* The migration and proliferation of connective tissue cells leading to 'scar' formation
2. *Regeneration.* The migration and proliferation of specialised cells re-establishing the anatomical and functional integrity of an organ or tissue.

These processes may act alone, but are usually found in combination.

MAJOR CAUSES OF TISSUE DESTRUCTION
1. Inflammatory agents
   (i) By direct physical or toxic effects
   (ii) Indirectly as a result of the host response, e.g. necrosis in tuberculosis
2. Traumatic excision
   (i) Accidental
   (ii) Surgical
3. Loss of blood supply

REPAIR
Repair involves two overlapping processes:
1. Organisation
2. Progressive fibrosis

1. *Organisation* is the conversion of dead tissue or inert material into *granulation tissue*—immature fibrovascular tissue. It is seen in:
   (i) Haematomas in wound and fracture healing
   (ii) Thrombi
   (iii) Infarcts
   (iv) Fibrinous exudates

Granulation tissue is formed by:
   (i) Migration of
      a. Undifferentiated connective tissue cells which swell and divide forming activated fibroblasts
      b. Macrophages which remove fibrin, red blood cells, etc.

(ii) Proliferation of endothelial cells forming capillary buds some of which fuse and differentiate into arterioles, capillaries and venules

(iii) Production of acid mucopolysaccharide ground substance by fibroblasts

(iv) Secretion of tropocollagen by more mature (bipolar) fibroblasts

(v) Aggregation of tropocollagen to form collagen fibrils

2. *Progressive fibrosis*

(i) Orientation and development of cross-linkages between collagen fibrils yields fibres with greater tensile strength

(ii) Reduction in vascularity

(iii) Conversion of fibroblasts to resting fibrocytes

(iv) Diminished cellularity

(v) Formation of an avascular, hypocellular scar

Further changes in scars:

(i) Cicatrisation—a late diminution in size producing deformity, e.g. hour-glass stomach following peptic ulceration

(ii) Calcification

(iii) Ossification

REGENERATION

The capacity of damaged tissues to respond by regeneration varies considerably. Three categories are generally recognised:

1. Labile cells which continue to proliferate throughout life, e.g. haemopoietic cells and enteroblasts of the small intestine

2. Stable cells which retain the capacity to proliferate, e.g. liver, kidney tubule cells, endocrine cells

3. Permanent cells which cannot reproduce themselves after birth, e.g. nervous system, cardiac muscle, complex sensory organs such as eyes and ears

Labile tissues heal by regeneration with little or no repair.

Permanent tissues are incapable of regeneration and heal entirely by repair. Most organs show evidence of both processes.

WOUND HEALING

In considering the healing of a skin wound, two types are usually distinguished:

1. A clean wound with a minimum of space between the margins—i.e. an incised wound

2. An open or excised wound

There are no fundamental differences in healing between these two categories, they merely differ in the degree to which the various stages apply.

1. *Stages in healing of an incised wound*
    (i)   Escape of blood and exudate
    (ii)   Acute inflammation during the first 24 h
    (iii) Proliferation and migration of epithelial cells of the epidermis which undermine the superficial blood clot forming a 'scab'. This regeneration is usually complete 24 to 36 h after injury
    (iv) Migration and proliferation of fibroblasts and endothelial cells (organisation) is seen between 48 and 72 h
    (v)   Appearance of thin branching bundles of collagen fibrils coated with ground substance (reticulin fibres) 4 to 5 days after injury
    (vi) Progressive increase in mature collagen fibres during the second week forming a scar
    (vii) Loss of vascularity and shrinkage of the scar

2. *Stages in healing of an excised wound*
    (i)   Filling of the wound by blood clot
    (ii)   Hardening of the surface forming a scab
    (iii) Acute inflammatory reaction
    (iv) Proliferation of epithelial cells which insinuate beneath the hard scab. Regeneration ceases when the cells meet in the centre of the wound probably as a result of 'contact inhibition' which arrests further movement and mitotic activity and may be mediated by chalones
    (v)   Organisation of the base and margins of the clot with the formation of granulation tissue
    (vi) Contraction of the wound; an early diminution in size considerably reducing the amount of tissue required for healing. The causes of contraction are not known but possible mechanisms are:
        a. Shrinkage of the scab in superficial wounds
        b. Contractile properties of granulation tissue attributable to contraction of fibroblasts or tissue re-modelling
    (vii) Epidermal thickening and further stimulation
    (viii) Progressive fibrosis
    (ix) Loss of vascularity and cicatrisation of the fibrous scar
Excised wound healing differs from incised in:
1. Greater tissue loss
2. More inflammatory exudate and necrotic material to remove
3. More granulation tissue therefore a bigger scar and more deformity
4. Wound contraction necessary
6. Slower process
7. Increased liability to infection

Factors influencing wound healing

1. *Local factors adversely affecting healing*
    (i)   Type of wounding agent; blunt, crushing, tearing etc.
    (ii)   Infection
    (iii) Foreign bodies in wound
    (iv)   Poor blood supply
    (v)   Excessive movement
    (vi)   Poor apposition of margins, e.g. large haematoma formation
    (vii) Poor wound contraction due to tissue tethering, e.g. skin over tibia
    (viii) Infiltration by tumour
    (ix)   Previous irradiation

2. *General factors adversely affecting healing*
    (i)   Poor nutrition
        a. Deficiency of protein. This results in a lack of the sulphur-containing amino acids methionine and cystine which are essential to the synthesis of collagen
        b. Lack of ascorbic acid (vitamin C) results in abnormal granulation tissue and deficient collagen production
    (ii)   Excessive glucocorticosteroid production or administration
    (iii) Fall in temperature
    (iv)   Jaundice

3. *Factors accelerating wound healing*
    (i)   Ultraviolet light
    (ii)   Administration of anabolic steroids, deoxycorticosterone acetate, and (?) growth hormone
    (iii) Rise in temperature

Complications of wound healing
   1. Wound rupture
   2. Infection
   3. Implantation of epidermal cells giving rise to a keratin-filled epidermoid cyst
   4. Weak scars with possible development of incisional herniae
   5. Cicatrisation and deformity
   6. Keloid formation. The production of an elevated scar by excessive connective tissue proliferation and fibrosis
   7. Malignant change. The development of squamous carcinoma in old healed incisions is a recognised but rare complication

HEALING OF A FRACTURE

Steps in the healing of a fractured long bone are:

1. *Haemorrhage* from the highly vascular severed ends
2. *Inflammation*
3. *Invasion of the clot* by macrophages, fibroblasts, and endothelial cells—organisation
4. *Proliferation* of cells from the elevated or torn periosteum and the endosteum lining the bone trabeculae. These differentiate in two directions,
   (i)   into chondroblasts which secrete sulphated mucopolysaccharides and collagen forming cartilage, and seen mainly when fracture is not fully immobilised
   (ii) into osteoblasts which secrete osseomucin and lay down irregular collagen fibres in trabeculae—so called *osteoid*
5. *Calcification* of cartilage and osteoid. The calcified osteoid is now termed non-lamellar or 'woven' bone. The hard fusiform mass linking the bone ends is fracture *'callus'*
6. *Removal of calcified cartilage and osteoid* by osteoclasts with simultaneous osteoblastic activity laying down orderly collagen plates with regular Haversian systems to form lamellar bone
7. *Remodelling* of the lamellar bone with strengthening along the lines of stress and removal of unwanted bone

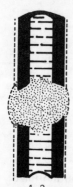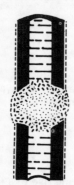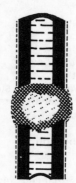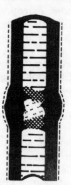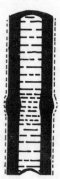

1, 2	3, 4	5	6	7
Haemorrhage Inflammation	Organisation Proliferation of periosteal cells	Woven bone and cartilage	Conversion to lamellar bone	Remodelling

Complications of fracture healing

1. Delayed union
2. Mal-union
   (i)   Angulation
   (ii) Shortening

3. Fibrous union resulting from
    (i)   Excessive movement which may lead to the development
           of a false joint (pseudoarthrosis)
    (ii)   Infection which may also give rise to osteomyelitis
    (iii) Ischaemia
4. Non-union if soft-tissues such as muscle or fat are
    interposed between the severed ends.

HEALING IN OTHER SITES

1. *Liver*
    (i)   After a single, short-lived injury such as drug-induced
           necrosis or acute hepatitis, the liver heals completely by
           regeneration
    (ii)   Repeated injury, as in alcoholic abuse or chronic
           hepatitis, leads to collapse of the reticulin framework,
           production of collagen by mesenchymal cells, and
           irregular, nodular regeneration, resulting in cirrhosis

2. *Kidney*
Regeneration is virtually confined to the tubular epithelium and is
seen for example after acute tubular necrosis. Otherwise injury
results in loss of glomeruli and scarring.

3. *Mucosal surfaces*
    (i)   Superficial ulceration is followed by regeneration of the
           epithelium but there may be loss of specialised cells. In
           the stomach, for example, healed areas may be covered
           by intestinal-type epithelium
    (ii)   Deeper ulceration with involvement of submucosa and
           muscle heals by scar formation and epithelial
           regeneration.

4. *Nervous system*
Adult nerve cells are incapable of mitotic division but limited
regeneration is possible
    (i)   Peripheral nerve section results in distal Wallerian
           degeneration, growth of axon-sprouts from the cut-end,
           and proliferation of Schwann cells, with eventual
           enclosure in a new myelin sheath
    (ii)   Central nervous system. If the involved nerve cell
           survives axons and dendrites can regrow, but most
           tissue loss is followed by astrocytic proliferation with the
           formation of a glial scar often around a fluid filled cavity

5. *Muscle*
- (i)   Cardiac muscle shows no regeneration and healing is achieved entirely by fibrous repair
- (ii) Skeletal muscle shows a limited capacity to regenerate and if only part of a muscle fibre is destroyed then the fibre may regrow within the sarcolemmal sheath
- (iii) Smooth muscle cells are capable of proliferation and minor tissue loss may be followed by successful regeneration

FURTHER READING

Iversen, O.H. (1973) The chalones. *Acta Pathologica et Microbiologica Scandinavica,* Suppl. **236**, 71.

Jayson, M.I.V. (Ed.) (1976) The fibrotic process: Symposium. *Annals of the Rheumatic Diseases,* **36**, Suppl. 2.

Longacre, J.J. (Ed.) (1976) Various aspects of wound healing. In *The Ultrastructure of Collagen.* Springfield, Ill.: Thomas.

Winstanley, E.W. (1974) Changes in epithelial thickness during the healing of excised full-thickness skin wounds. *Journal of Pathology,* **114**, 155.

Chronic inflammation

'A process in which there is continuing inflammation at the same time as attempts at healing resulting from persistence of the injurious agent'.

Mechanisms
1. Defective acute inflammatory response
   (i) Poor blood supply
   (ii) Poor general nutrition
   (iii) Abnormal neutrophil function
   (iv) Anti-inflammatory drugs, especially corticosteroids
2. Delayed hypersensitivity reactions and auto-immune disease
   (i) Intracellular infectious agents, e.g. tuberculosis, salmonellosis, brucellosis, viral infections
   (ii) Repeated contact sensitivity, e.g. contact dermatitis to rubber, nickel, etc.
   (iii) Auto-immune diseases, e.g. diffuse lymphocytic thyroiditis (Hashimoto's disease), auto-immune gastritis
3. Foreign-body reactions. These act as a nidus for persistent infection or as tissue irritants which directly provoke a chronic inflammatory reaction. Such irritants can be divided into:
   (i) Endogenous, e.g. necrotic adipose tissue, cholesterol crystals, uric acid crystals in gout
   (ii) Exogenous, e.g. suture material, metallic fragments, silica, asbestos fibres

CLASSIFICATION
1. Clinical
   (i) Following a recognisable acute inflammation, e.g. chronic osteomyelitis
   (ii) Arising *de novo*, e.g. brucellosis, tuberculosis

2. Histological
   (i) Specific—having a reproducible histological pattern, e.g. tuberculosis, syphilis, leprosy.
   (ii) Non-specific—showing only the general features of inflammation, e.g. chronic cholecystitis, chronic pyelonephritis

GENERAL FEATURES
1. Continuing acute inflammation
    (i)   Increased vascularity
    (ii) Polymorph infiltration
    (iii) Fibrinous exudate
2. Phagocytosis by macrophages of cell debris, and the injurious agent in some circumstances. Where macrophages are the predominant cell, and are found in circumscribed aggregates (granulomata) the inflammatory reaction is termed 'granulomatous'
3. Features of healing—repair and/or regeneration
4. Infiltration by lymphocytes and plasma cells—'chronic inflammatory cells'

CELLS OF CHRONIC INFLAMMATION
A. Macrophages
1. *The mononuclear phagocyte system*
A system composed of macrophages and their precursors.
Macrophages are characterised by:
    (i)   Marked phagocytic activity—capable of ingesting large particles such as red blood cells, protozoa, etc. as well as bacteria
    (ii) Firm attachment when exposed to a glass surface
    (iii) Ruffling of outer (plasma) membrane under EM

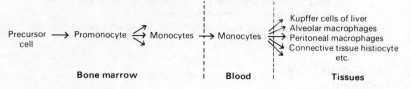

Precursor cell → Promonocyte ⇄ Monocytes → Monocytes → Kupffer cells of liver / Alveolar macrophages / Peritoneal macrophages / Connective tissue histiocyte etc.

Bone marrow   **Blood**   **Tissues**

2. *Functions*
Phagocytosis of cell debris after necrosis
Ingestion and storage of irritant substances, e.g. carbon particles
Ingestion and destruction of bacteria (particularly after lymphokine response)
Antigen trapping and concentration at the cell surface
Phagocytosis and processing of antigen with production of fragments (coupled with RNA?) which are highly immunogenic
Synthesis of complement components
Synthesis of interferon
Synthesis of a Macrophage Mitogenic Factor (?)
Limitation of the spread of viral infections (not interferon mediated)
Persistence of viruses in macrophages may be important in long-lasting immunity following some viral infections
Release of various enzymes (lysozyme, plasminogen activator, collagenase and elastase) which bring about lysis of extracellular fibrin, collagen and elastin

3. *Chemotaxis*
The following agents have been shown to have chemotactic activity for macrophages *in vitro:*
  (i)   Monocyte chemotactic factor (lymphokine)
  (ii) Antigen/antibody complexes in plasma
  (iii) Plasmin + serum

4. *Special forms of macrophages*
  (i)   Epithelioid cells—epithelial-like eosinophilic macrophages showing diminished phagocytosis seen in tuberculosis, sarcoidosis, Crohn's granulomata, etc.
  (ii) Siderophages—haemosiderin-laden macrophages seen after haemorrhage in chronic venous congestion of the lung ('heart-failure cells'), haemosiderosis, etc.
  (iii) Melanophages—melanin containing macrophages seen in the interstices of a malignant melanoma, in the dermis in certain forms of chronic dermatitis, etc.
  (iv) Lipophages—macrophages with 'ground glass' cytoplasm after phagocytosis of altered fat, e.g. in traumatic fat necrosis

5. *Giant cells*
In some circumstances macrophages fuse and give rise to multinucleate giant-cells:
  (i)   Infections, e.g. tuberculosis (Langhan's cell), fungal infections, syphilis
  (ii) Foreign-body reactions
  (iii) Phagocytosis of lipid (Touton giant-cells) in xanthomata, dermatofibroma, etc.
  (iv) Collagen diseases, e.g. rheumatic fever (Aschoff giant-cells), rheumatoid nodules
  (v)   Unknown aetiology, e.g. sarcoidosis, Crohn's disease

B. Eosinophils
Whilst eosinophils are seen in certain acute inflammatory responses such as atopic hypersensitivity reactions, they are more characteristic of chronic inflammation.

1. *Functions* (possible)
  (i)   Neutralisation of histamine and 5-HT
  (ii) Processing of antigen
  (iii) Phagocytosis of antigen-antibody complexes

2. Chemotaxis

Eosinophils respond to the same chemotactic factors as neutrophil polymorphs with the following important additions:

(i) Eosinophil chemotactic factor of anaphylaxis (ECF-A) released from sensitised tissues on exposure to antigen

(ii) A specific eosinophil chemotactic factor produced by sensitised T-lymphocytes on exposure to antigen

(iii) A pre-formed factor released from mast-cell granules (ECF-M) which may be identical with ECF-A

(iv) A complement dependent factor found in guinea-pig serum, ECF-C

C. Lymphocytes and plasma cells

Small lymphocytes can be divided into two reactive populations:

(i) T-lymphocytes, which are thymus dependent and are responsible for cellular immunity

(ii) B-lymphocytes, which are processed by tissue equivalent to the bursa of Fabricius of chickens (possibly gut-associated lymphoid tissue) and are responsible for humoral (antibody-mediated) immunity

On contact with the appropriate antigen both types of sensitised small lymphocytes undergo blast-cell transformation, the B-cells developing into plasma cells which actively secrete the corresponding antibody, and the T-cells producing a number of soluble factors—lymphokines, important in mediating chronic inflammation. There is co-operation between T-cells and macrophages in the recognition, concentration and processing of certain antigens prior to a B-cell response.

A third population is composed of unreactive lymphocytes which have been designated 'null-cells'.

1. Role of antibodies in chronic inflammation

(i) Opsonisation of bacteria prior to phagocytosis by macrophages

(ii) Neutralisation of toxins

(iii) Formation of antigen – antibody complexes which activate the complement sequence

2. Lymphokines

These are variable m.wt. (20000 to 80000) moieties released by sensitised T-cells on contact with antigen. They function as an amplification system in the cellular immune response and have the following actions:

(i) Recruitment of macrophages
   a. Monocyte Chemotactic Factor (MCF)
   b. Macrophage Migration Inhibition Factor (MIF)
   c. Macrophage Activation and Arming factors enhance killing of phagocytosed bacteria or of target cells

(ii)   *Mediation of inflammatory response*
    a. Skin reactive factor initiates cell migration and increased vascular permeability when injected into the skin of non-sensitised animals
    b. Eosinophil chemotactic factor

(iii) *Recruitment of other lymphocytes*
    a. Lymphocyte transforming factor permits non-sensitised lymphocytes to be stimulated by antigen
    b. Lymphocyte mitogenic factor stimulates other lymphocytes directly in the absence of antigen
    c. Transfer factor consists of a short polypeptide chain joined to 3 or 4 RNA bases which can confer on previously unresponsive recipients the capacity to mount delayed hypersensitivity skin reactions to a variety of microbial antigens

(iv)   *Effects on target cells*
    a. Lymphotoxin—a soluble toxic factor that may be responsible for lymphocyte-mediated destruction of tissues.
    b. Macrophage cytotoxic factor

(v)   *Production of interferon*
    a. As a result of direct stimulation of lymphocyte synthesis by viruses
    b. Macrophage synthesis may be enhanced by lymphokines

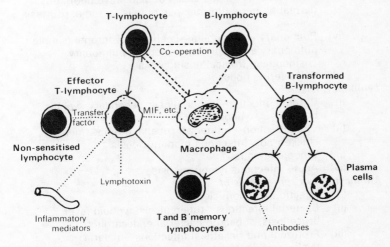

Responses of sensitised lymphocytes to antigen

GENERAL RESPONSES TO INFLAMMATION

1. *Pyrexia* resulting from the effects on the temperature regulation centre in the hypothalamus of:
- (i)   Bacterial pyrogens
- (ii) Endogenous pyrogens derived from polymorphs and macrophages

2. *Negative nitrogen balance*

3. *Increased erythrocyte sedimentation rate*

4. *Anaemia* as a result of:
- (i)   Blood loss from inflammatory lesions
- (ii) Haemolysis
- (iii) Toxic depression of the bone marrow

5. *Leucocytosis:*
Neutrophilia in
- (i)   Pyogenic infections
- (ii) Tissue breakdown—myocardial infarction, mesenteric infarction

Eosinophilia in
- (i)   Allergic disorders—hay fever, drug allergy
- (ii) Parasitic infestation—trichinosis, schistosomiasis, filariasis, hydatid disease, strongyloides
- (iii) Skin diseases—some cases of exfoliative dermatitis, dermatitis herpetiformis, pemphigus, eczema, psoriasis, scabies
- (iv) Pulmonary eosinophilia—Loeffler's syndrome (simple pulmonary eosinophilia), prolonged pulmonary eosinophilia, tropical eosinophilia
- (v)   Polyarteritis nodosa

Lymphocytosis in
- (i)   Chronic infection—tuberculosis, secondary syphilis brucellosis, typhoid fever
- (ii) Viral infection—influenza, rubella, mumps, measles, chicken-pox, infectious mononucleosis
- (iii) Whooping-cough
- (iv) Acute infectious lymphocytosis

Monocytosis in some cases of
- (i)   Infectious mononucleosis
- (ii) Bacterial infections—tuberculosis, typhoid fever, brucellosis, subacute bacterial endocarditis
- (iii) Protozoal and rickettsial infections—malaria, leishmaniasis, trypanosomiasis, Rocky Mountain spotted fever

6. *Reactive hyperplasia of the reticuloendothelial and lymphoid systems* (especially with chronic inflammation)
   (i)   Enlargement of regional lymph nodes
   (ii) Hepatomegaly (and 'non-specific reactive hepatitis')
   (iii) Splenomegaly

7. *Degenerative changes* in other organs as a result of persistent 'toxaemia', e.g. fatty change and hydropic vacuolation in the liver

8. *Constitutional symptoms*—malaise, anorexia, headache, loss of weight, etc.

FURTHER READING

Adams, D.O. (1976) The granulomatous inflammatory response. *American Journal of Pathology,* **84,** 163.

British Journal of Haematology (1976) Annotation: functions of the eosinophil leucocyte. *British Journal of Haematology,* **33,** 313.

Dvorak, A.M., Dvorak, H.F., Mihm, M.C., Jr., Johnson, R.A., Manseau, E.J., Morgan, E. & Colvin, R.B. (1974) Morphology of delayed-type hypersensitivity reactions in man: quantitative description of the inflammatory response. *Laboratory Investigation,* **31,** 111.

Dvorak, A.M., Dvorak, H.F. & Mihm, M.C. Jr (1976) Morphology of delayed type hypersensitivity response in man: ultrastructural alterations affecting the microvasculature and the tissue mast cells. *Laboratory Investigation,* **34,** 179.

Nelson, D.S. (Ed.) (1976) *Immunobiology of the Macrophage.* London: Academic Press.

Immunopathology

The immune system is concerned with the recognition of foreign materials (*antigens*) and through a variety of reactions rejecting or nullifying them. In carrying out these functions the system must be capable of distinguishing foreign, that is 'non-self', from 'self'. In the fetus the developing lymphoid system is exposed to body constituents and is rendered unresponsive (*tolerant*) to these self proteins. When immunological maturity is established after the neonatal period, a non-self protein is recognised as foreign and a specific immunological reaction follows. There are two basic types of reaction:

1. The formation of immunoglobulins which are released into the blood and other body fluids—humoral antibodies
2. The production of specifically sensitised small lymphocytes which possess antibody-like molecules on their surface and are the effectors of cell-mediated immunity

Tolerance to foreign antigens can be established by introducing them into the body during fetal or neonatal development whereafter they are accepted as self. In the adult, tolerance can be induced with very low doses of antigen (by affecting T-cells), while high doses may render both T- and B-cells unresponsive. It seems likely that T- and B-cells cooperate in maintaining tolerance towards the body's own constituents. Tolerance may be reinforced by *suppressor* T-cells which prevent reactions to self proteins. When this state of tolerance breaks down, the immune system may produce antibodies or mount a cell-mediated attack directed against self constituents—*auto-immunity*. Such adverse, auto-aggressive reactions are one aspect of *allergy* or *hypersensitivity*. These are immunological reactions to an antigen which produce detrimental results.

THE IMMUNE RESPONSE

A. Primary response

When antigen comes into contact with a genetically 'programmed' responsive small lymphocyte, the cell reacts by enlarging, becoming pyroninophilic, and exhibiting mitotic activity—*blast-cell transformation*. These immunoblasts may:

1. Develop rough endoplasmic reticulum and differentiate into plasma cells which manufacture a specific antibody
2. Proliferate to produce a population (*clone*) of cells capable of acting as an effector cell in a specific cell-mediated response
3. Revert to a lymphocytic form and act as a primed 'memory' cell

B. Secondary response

On subsequent exposure to the same antigen, there is some interaction with pre-formed humoral antibody and with an enlarged population of responsive lymphocytes. There is therefore a greatly amplified humoral antibody response and a more rapid recruitment of sensitised cells.

IMMUNOGLOBULINS

Immunoglobulins share a similar basic structure. They consist of two heavy and two light polypeptide chains linked by disulphide bonds. Splitting by papain produces two univalent fragments capable of binding antigen (Fab) and a third fragment without this capacity (Fc fragment).

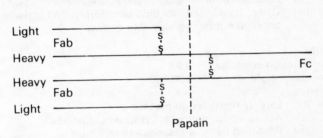

The light chains are of two types, kappa (κ) and lambda (λ) and each immunoglobulin molecule has either two κ or two λ chains but never one of each. The heavy chains are of 5 major types and each molecule has a pair of identical type. Thus five distinct immunoglobulin classes are recognised on the basis of their heavy chains: IgG, IgA, IgM, IgD and IgE.

1. IgG

Sedimentation coefficient = 7S
Molecular weight   = 150 000
Properties:

- (i)   Crosses the placental barrier and is therefore the major protective immunoglobulin in the neonate
- (ii) Diffuses easily into all extracellular fluids
- (iii) Acts as an antitoxin (neutralising antibody)
- (iv) Responsible for opsonic binding of bacteria
- (v)   Coats cells prior to killing by K-cells. (Macrophages and lymphocytes with specific cytotoxic activity)
- (vi) Complement fixation

2. IgA

Exists as monomer, dimers, trimers, and polymers so that the sedimentation coefficient ranges from 7S to 11S. It polymerises by spontaneous binding through a cysteine-rich polypeptide (J-chain)

Molecular weight   = 160000+

Properties:

(i)   Principal immunoglobulin in secretions such as those of the respiratory and gastrointestinal tracts and in sweat, saliva, tears, and colostrum

(ii) Produced locally and secreted as the dimer bound to a third polypeptide, the secretory or transport piece, which stabilises the molecule against proteolysis

(iii) Prevents infection of mucous membranes by inhibiting adhesion of organisms to the epithelium

(iv) When aggregated will bind polymorphs and activate complement by the alternate pathway

3. IgM

Sedimentation coefficient = 19S

Molecular weight   = 900000

Properties:

(i)   Largely restricted to plasma

(ii) Act as agglutinating or cytotoxic antibodies

(iii) Produced early in response to infection

4. IgD

Sedimentation coefficient = 7S

Molecular weight   = 185000

Properties:

(i)   ? acts as a cytophilic antibody on lymphocytes in the neonate

5. IgE

Sedimentation coefficient = 8S

Molecular weight   = 200000

Properties:

(i)   Becomes firmly fixed to skin and to mast cells. These coated cells degranulate when exposed to the appropriate antigen and release histamine and other agents

HYPERSENSITIVITY

Excessive or altered reactions to an antigen producing adverse effects are termed hypersensitivity or allergy. These reactions have been classified into five groups:

Type I—Immediate (anaphylactic-type) hypersensitivity

Type II—Cytotoxic type hypersensitivity

Type III—Complex-mediated hypersensitivity

Type IV—Delayed-type (cell-mediated) hypersensitivity

Type V—Stimulatory hypersensitivity

Type I—Anaphylactic

A. Systemic anaphylaxis

Anaphylactic shock is characterised by intense bronchospasm, laryngeal oedema and a fall in blood pressure, and occasionally results in death. It can be provoked by injecting a large dose of an antigen some time after one or more smaller sensitising doses of the same antigen. The principal pathogenetic type is *Cytotrophic* anaphylaxis where antigen reacts with antibodies (usually of the IgE class) bound to mast cells or basophils by their Fc portions and results in the release of vasoactive amines. Anaphylaxis can also result from Type III reactions (see below)

B. Local anaphylaxis (atopic allergy)

Local reactions result from the exposure of tissue mast cells in sensitised individuals to specific antigens and are seen in 3 main situations:

1. Respiratory tract
   (i)   Allergic rhinitis (hay fever)
   (ii) Extrinsic asthma
2. Intestine: Food allergy—shellfish, strawberries etc
3. Skin: Urticarial reactions to drugs, chemicals, injected antigens, etc.

In highly sensitised individuals provocation with the appropriate antigen may result in systemic anaphylaxis.

Type II—Cytotoxic

Reactions of this type occur when an antibody combines with an antigen on the surface of a cell and results in cell-death by:

   (i)   Complement-mediated cytolysis (C89)
   (ii) Phagocytosis of the cell in response to an opsonic antibody effect or by immune adherence (C3)
   (iii) Promotion of K-cell cytotoxicity

Examples:

   (i)   Haemolysis resulting from antibodies directed against red-cell antigens or antigens attached to the surface
         a. Transfusion reactions
         b. Rhesus incompatability
         c. Auto-immune haemolytic anaemia
         d. Drug-induced haemolysis, e.g. α-methyldopa, chlorpromazine, phenacetin
         e. Associated infections, e.g. salmonellosis
   (ii) Thrombocytopenia following treatment with Sedormid (now withdrawn) and occasionally with aspirin, tetracyclines, PAS, oestrogen and other drugs
   (iii) Agranulocytosis associated with amidopyrine, quinine, PAS, thiouracil, colchicine, phenothiazines, etc.
   (iv) Anti-glomerular basement membrane antibodies in Goodpasture's syndrome activate complement and provoke an acute inflammatory response in the glomerulus

Type III—Complex-mediated

When antigen and antibody react in the presence of an excess of antigen the complexes so formed are soluble and may be carried in the circulation to sites distant from their source. Such complexes are deposited in capillary plexuses and are therefore found in the renal glomeruli, the skin, the intestine, in synovial membranes etc. When complexes are formed in antibody excess they tend to be insoluble and remain localised to the site of formation. Complexes of this type entering the circulation are cleared rapidly by macrophages of the RES.

Antigen-antibody complexes will initiate an *acute inflammatory reaction* by the activation of complement and subsequent formation of anaphylotoxins, leucotoxins, and aggregation of platelets. *Tissue destruction* may result from complement-mediated cytolysis or by release of lysosomal enzymes from polymorphs which will also activate factor XII and promote *coagulation*.

A. *Antibody excess*

(i)   Arthus reation—an acute vasculitis produced by the introduction of antigen into the skin in the presence of high levels of precipitating antibody (IgG), e.g.
  a. Reaction to insulin injection in sensitised diabetics
  b. Erythema nodosum leprosum

(ii) In the lung (allergic alveolitis)
  a. Farmer's lung—Type III reaction to *Micropolyspora faeni*
  b. Bird fancier's lung—(?) reaction to avian proteins in droppings
  c. Hypersensitivity to *Aspergillus fumigatus*
  d. Maple bark-stripper's disease
  e. Mushroom-picker's lung
  f. Paprika-splitter's lung
  g. Bagassosis (burnt sugar cane)

B. *Antigen excess*

The classical example of this form of complex deposition is 'serum sickness'—a syndrome characterised by pyrexia, urticaria, joint pains, generalised lymphadenopathy and albuminuria, which is occasionally seen following large injections of foreign protein. Other examples of immune complex disease are:

(i)   Glomerulonephritis
  a. Post-streptococcal and other infections
  b. Systemic lupus erythematosus (SLE)
  c. Quartan malaria
  d. Drug-induced, e.g. penicillamine in rheumatoid arthritis

(ii) Skin lesions
  a. Erythema multiforme
  b. Secondary syphilis

(iii) 'Vasculitides'
  a. Polyarteritis nodosa (?)

   b. Henoch-Schönlein disease
   c. Drug-induced vasculitis
   d. Wegener's granulomatosis (?)
(iv) Lung lesions due to such complexes occur in
   a. Respiratory syncitial virus infection
   b. Measles in an 'immunised' individual
(v) Central Nervous system
   a. SLE
(vi) Arthritis (associated with various viral infections)
(vii) Rheumatic fever (complexes with streptococcal antigen deposited in small blood vessels in a wide variety of tissues)

Type IV—Delayed-type hypersensitivity

Delayed hypersensitivity is mediated by T-lymphocytes. When a sensitised T-lymphocyte (T-memory cell) comes into contact with the appropriate antigen it undergoes blast-cell transformation and cell-division. Simultaneously, the cell produces numerous soluble factors—lymphokines, which promote a mixed inflammatory reaction (see p. 32). T-lymphocyte responses are usually beneficial and underlie a number of important defence mechanisms against certain bacterial, viral and fungal infections (cell-mediated immunity). In some circumstances however they may have a deleterious effect and constitute a hypersensitivity reaction
Examples:
   (i)   Cell-mediated hypersensitivity to bacterial antigens (bacterial allergy) is responsible for:
      a. The Mantoux reaction to an intradermal injection of tuberculin
      b. Caseation in tuberculosis
      c. The tuberculoid form of leprosy
   (ii) Contact hypersensitivity in the skin: simple chemicals acting as haptens attach to skin proteins and render them antigenic. The resulting cell-mediated response produces erythema, oedema and often vesiculation—contact dermatitis. Common skin sensitisers are:
      a. Nickel
      b. Rubber
      c. Poison-ivy and primulas
      d. Topical medicaments—neomycin, lanolin, penicillin
      e. Iodine
      f. Dinitrochlorobenzene (DNCB)
   (iii) Homograft rejection
   (iv) Some auto-immune diseases

Type V—Stimulatory hypersensitivity

Thus far only one example of this form of hypersensitivity has been defined and that is the stimulatory auto-antibody responsible for a type of thyrotoxicosis (Graves' disease). The auto-antibody, long-acting thyroid stimulator (LATS), is directed at the same surface antigenic site as is activated by TSH, and results in prolonged hypersecretion of thyroxine and triiodothyronine by the cell.

TISSUE TRANSPLANTATION

Nomenclature
Autograft—transplantation within the same individual
Isograft or syngeneic graft—between identical twins or in-bred animals
Allograft—between individuals of differing genetic make-up (formerly homograft)
Xenograft—between different species

Transplantation antigens
All nucleated cells possess surface histocompatibility antigens determined by separate gene loci. There is one major system, the HL-A antigens, and over 30 have been identified. Tests for histocompatibility employ leucocytes and the specific antisera. Although an individual's tissues are antigenically similar, the concentration of antigens varies from tissue to tissue, for example skin has a high concentration, whilst placenta, muscle, aortic wall, have low levels.

Rejection
Three patterns are described:
(i)   Hyperacute rejection occurs where there is major incompatibility with high levels of humoral antibodies resulting in an Arthus-type reaction
(ii) Acute rejection occurs 2 to 3 weeks after grafting and results from cell-mediated hypersensitivity. Destruction of the graft is brought about by:
  a. The direct action of sensitised 'killer' T-lymphocytes
  b. Phagocytosis of graft cells by activated macrophages (by MAF)
  c. Attack by K-cells on IgG-coated graft cells
(iii) Chronic rejection consequent upon gradual vascular obliteration, probably due to deposition of immune complexes and activation of complement and blood coagulation

Prevention of rejection
(i)   Favourable sites for transplantation
  a. Cornea and anterior chamber of the eye
  b. Meninges
  c. Testis
  These sites may be protected by virtue of unusual vascularity or lymphatic drainage.
(ii) Accurate tissue matching
(iii) Immune deficiency states, pregnancy, and uraemia
(iv) Immunosuppression
  a. Corticosteroids
  b. Azathioprine
  c. Antilymphocyte serum
  d. Whole-body irradiation
  e. Induction of immune tolerance

AUTO-IMMUNITY

Mechanisms

The formation of antibodies or cell-mediated reactions directed against 'self' constituents may result from:

1. *Alteration of self-proteins*
   (i)   Combination with haptens, as in contact dermatitis and α-methyldopa-induced haemolysis
   (ii) Modification by degenerative or infective conditions e.g. to skin proteins following burns, red cells in mycoplasma infection.

2. *Hidden antigens*
   Some antigens remain hidden or sequestered from the immune system and tolerance does not develop. On subsequent exposure in the mature animal they will be treated as non-self.
   (i)   Spermatozoa. Orchitis may be followed by production of antisperm antibodies and lead to sterility
   (ii) Lens protein. Degeneration and/or removal of a cataract may result in auto-antibodies and damage to the contralateral lens

3. *Cross-reactions*
   Immune reactions to exogenous antigen may cross-react with self-proteins
   (i)   Antibodies to streptococcal antigens may react with constituents of cardiac muscle or connective tissue in rheumatic fever
   (ii) An immune response to heterologous brain tissue in rabies vaccine may give rise to encephalitis

4. *Breakdown of tolerance*
   (i)   Genetic. An inherited defect or lack of efficiency in antibody production may lead to the formation of damaging antigen-excess complexes
   (ii) Direct disturbance of the immune system by drugs, chemicals, infective agents, and neoplasia. Examples:
        a. Hydralazine precipitating SLE
        b. *Mycobacterium tuberculosis* promotes auto-immune reactions (as in Freund's complete adjuvant)
        c. Virus infection of NZB mice appears to underlie the development of auto-immune haemolytic anaemia and complex-mediated glomerulonephritis
        d. Chronic lymphatic leukaemia and malignant lymphomas may be associated with auto-immune haemolytic anaemia.

Pathogenesis of auto-immune disease

Auto-antibodies can be found in the sera of apparently healthy individuals and increase in incidence with age. In most cases no harmful effects can be attributed to the antibodies. Auto-immune reactions having a primary role in disease operate through:

1. Humoral antibodies in
   (i)   Auto-immune haemolytic anaemia
   (ii)   Idiopathic thrombocytopenia
   (iii)   Some cases of lymphopenia
   (iv)   Some cases of agranulocytosis
   (v)   Hashimoto's thyroiditis (anti-thyroglobulin, anti-microsomal)—?
   (vi)   Pernicious anaemia (anti-intrinsic factor, anti-parietal cell)
   (vii)   Some cases of male infertility (anti-spermatozoa)
   (viii) Goodpasture's syndrome
   (ix)   Lens-induced endophthalmitis
   (x)   Thyrotoxicosis (stimulatory)
2. Immune complexes in
   (i)   SLE (anti-DNA)
   (ii)   NZB mice infected with leukaemia virus
   (iii)   Aleutian mink disease
3. Cell-mediated reactions in
   (i)   Experimental allergic encephalomyelitis
           and in association with auto-antibodies in
   (ii)   Atrophic gastritis
   (iii)   Hashimoto's disease
   (iv)   Auto-immune orchitis

Diseases in which auto-antibodies are found but a primary role in producing the disease has not been established include:

1. Connective tissue disorders
   (i)   Rheumatoid disease—anti-IgG, anti-IgM antibody
   (ii)   Scleroderma—anti-IgG/antinuclear
   (iii)   Dermatomyositis—anti IgG/antinuclear
   (iv)   SLE—lymphocytoxic antibodies
2. Skin diseases
   (i)   Discoid lupus erythematosus—antinuclear/anti-IgG
   (ii)   Pemphigus—anti-intercellular cement substance
   (iii)   Pemphigoid—anti-basement membrane
   (iv)   Dermatitis herpetiformis—anti-reticulin
3. Alimentary system
   (i)   Ulcerative colitis/Crohn's disease—lymphocytotoxic
   (ii)   Primary biliary cirrhosis—antimitochondrial
   (iii)   Chronic active hepatitis—anti-smooth muscle
   (iv)   Some cases of 'cryptogenic' cirrhosis
4. Others
   (i)   Idiopathic adrenal cortical atrophy (Addison's disease)
   (ii)   Sjögren's syndrome
   (iii)   Multiple sclerosis
   (iv)   Myasthenia gravis (anti end-plate)
   (v)   Juvenile diabetes mellitus

IMMUNODEFICIENCY

The proper functioning of the immune system depends upon the integrity of the thymus, the bone marrow, and the gut-associated lymphoid tissues. Deficiencies in the system may result from a congenital defect in these tissues or secondarily to some other disease disturbing the normal function of the system.

A. Primary immunodeficiency
  1. Pure immunoglobulin deficiency
      (i)   Bruton-type agammaglobulinaemia
      (ii) Hypogammaglobulinaemia of late onset
      (iii) Dysgammaglobulinaemia
            a. IgG and IgA low, and IgM elevated
            b. IgA and IgM low, IgG is normal
            c. Isolated IgA deficiency (sometimes associated with intestinal nodular lymphoid hyperplasia, malabsorption, and Giardiasis)

In these disorders there is susceptibility to bacterial and yeast infections, but virus infections are controlled normally. Cell-mediated reactions are intact.

  2. Pure T-cell deficiency
      (i)   Thymic agenesis (Nezelof syndrome)
      (ii) Thymic alymphoplasia (dysplasia)
      (iii) Thymic hypoplasia or aplasia, absence of the parathyroids, and abnormalities of the aortic arch (Di George's syndrome) due to maldevelopment of the 3rd and 4th branchial arches

Here the immunoglobulin levels are normal but there is a complete absence of cell-mediated reactions.

  3. Mixed deficiency
      (i)   Stem-cell failure (reticular dysgenesis) results in a complete absence of white cells and lymphoid tissue
      (ii) Swiss-type agammaglobulinaemia—thymus and lymphoid tissues are hypoplastic
      (iii) Ataxia-telangiectasia syndrome
            a. Cerebellar ataxia
            b. Oculocutaneous telangiectasia
            c. Recurrent respiratory tract infections
            d. Low IgA and IgE
      (iv) Wiskott-Aldrich syndrome
            a. Atopic eczema
            b. Thrombocytopenia
            c. Recurrent infections
            d. Low IgM

B. Secondary immunodeficiency
Resulting from:
1. Excessive loss of immunoglobulins
   (i) Protein-losing enteropathy
   (ii) Nephrotic syndrome
2. Depression of the immune system by
   (i) Old age
   (ii) Malnutrition
   (iii) Virus infections such as measles
   (iv) Leprosy
   (v) Malaria
   (vi) Sarcoidosis
   (vii) Surgery
   (viii) Endotoxaemia
   (ix) Uraemia
3. Immunosuppression by
   (i) X-rays
   (ii) Corticosteroids
   (iii) Cytotoxic drugs
   (iv) Antilymphocyte serum
   (v) Antimetabolites
4. Neoplasia
   (i) Hodgkin's disease—T-cell deficiency

   (ii) Multiple myeloma $\left.\right\}$ deficiency of normal immunoglobulins
   (iii) Waldenström's macroglobulinaemia

   (iv) Non-Hodgkin's lymphoma $\left.\right\}$ mixed deficiency
   (v) Chronic lymphatic leukaemia
5. Splenectomy—diminished clearance of particulate antigens and impaired production of IgM antibodies
6. 'Idiopathic' splenic atrophy

FURTHER READING

Dequesnoy, R.J. & Abramoff, P. (1974) In *Pathologic Physiology,* 5th edn., ed. Sodeman, W.A. & Sodeman, W.A. p. 124. Philadelphia: Saunders.

Roitt, I.M. (1977) *Essential Immunology,* 3rd edn. Oxford: Blackwell.

Sell, S. (1975) *Immunology, Immunopathology and Immunity.* New York: Harper & Row.

Resistance to infection

Resistance to infection is dependent upon:
  A. The general body defence mechanisms
  B. Innate non-specific immunity
  C. Acquired specific immunity

A. BODY DEFENCES
  1. Physical barriers
    (i)   Skin
    (ii) Urothelium
    (iii) Mucous membranes of alimentary tract
  2. Mechanical decontamination
    (i)   Desquamation of surface cells together with adherent organisms
    (ii) Ciliary action
    (iii) Mucus trapping and expulsion
    (iv) Anatomical trapping, e.g. nasal turbinates
  3. Antimicrobial secretions
    (i)   Lysozyme (muramidase) in sweat, tears, saliva and tissue fluids
    (ii) Acidity of sweat, gastric juice and vaginal secretion
    (iii) Unsaturated fatty acids in sebum and sweat
    (iv) Immunoglobulins, e.g. IgA in intestinal secretions
  4. Surface phagocytosis by:
    (i)   Macrophages, e.g. alveolar macrophages
    (ii) Epithelial cells, e.g. in the bladder
  5. Competition by commensal organisms in:
    (i)   Upper respiratory tract
    (ii) Mouth
    (iii) Lower ileum and colon
    (iv) Vagina

B. INNATE IMMUNE MECHANISMS
  1. Genetic factors
    (i)   Species, e.g. animals are generally resistant to syphilis, poliomyelitis, meningococcal meningitis whereas humans are immune to myxomatosis, foot and mouth disease, etc.
    (ii) Race, e.g. Negroes and American Indians are more susceptible to tuberculosis than Caucasians
    (iii) Individual (hereditary factors)
    (iv) Sex. The male is more prone to fatal infectious disease than the female
    (v)   Age. The very young and the elderly are more susceptible to infection
    (vi) Hormonal status, e.g. infections are more common in diabetes mellitus, steroid therapy, hypothyroidism

  2. Cellular factors
      Phagocytosis by macrophages and polymorphs
  3. Humoral factors
    (i)   Lysozyme, is an enzyme which acts on the muramic acid present in bacterial cell walls
    (ii) Complement. Activation may bring about several antimicrobial effects:
        a. Bacteriolysis
        b. Opsonisation
        c. Immune adherence
        d. Leucotaxis
    (iii) Interferon, a non-specific antiviral agent produced by a wide variety of cells but particularly by cells of the RES in response to an inducer which is probably the nucleoprotein component of the virion. Interferon is more important in the elimination of viruses in non-immune individuals than in preventing infection
    (iv) 'Natural' opsonins

C. ACQUIRED IMMUNITY

Immunity based upon specific immunoglobulins either circulating or cell-bound to sensitised lymphocytes is *active* where an individual manufactures antibodies in response to an antigen, or *passive* where temporary protection is afforded by giving pre-formed antibodies.

  1. Active immunity
    (i) Natural, following previous infection
    (ii) Artificial, by administering toxoid, killed or attenuated organisms
        a. Toxoid, e.g. formaldehyde-treated exotoxin of diphtheria bacilli
        b. Killed organisms, e.g. typhoid vaccine, poliomyelitis (Salk) vaccine
        c. Attenuated organisms, e.g. Bacille-Calmette-Guérin vaccine is a live attenuated strain of *Mycobacterium tuberculosis*
  2. Passive immunity
    (i) Natural, transfer of antibodies of maternal origin
        a. Trans-placental
        b. Intestinal absorption from colostrum and milk
    (ii) Artificial, by the administration of immunoglobulins
        a. Homologous, e.g. pooled human gammaglobulin used in treatment of measles, hypogammaglobulinaemia, etc.
        b. Heterologous, e.g. tetanus anti-toxin prepared in the horse

IMMUNITY TO BACTERIAL INFECTION
1. Humoral factors
    (i)   Neutralising antibodies (anti-toxins) directed against bacterial exotoxins, e.g. antibodies against the erythrogenic exotoxin of *Streptococcus pyogenes* which gives rise to the skin changes of scarlet fever.
    (ii)   Opsonic antibodies which greatly enhance phagocytosis. Cytophilic antibodies may also contribute to the increased attachment of bacteria to the cell surface
    (iii) Activation of complement by specific antibodies combining with bacteria
    (iv)   Serum lysozyme
    (v)   Agglutinating antibodies may help localisation of infection
2. Cellular factors
    (i)   Lymphokine release by sensitised T-lymphocytes
    (ii)   Phagocytosis by polymorphs and macrophages
    (iii) Intracellular killing. Killing by macrophages is greatly enhanced following activation by the lymphokines MIF and MAF (see p. 32)
    (iv)   Macrophage processing of antigen and stimulation of B-lymphocyte response

IMMUNITY TO VIRAL INFECTION
1. Humoral factors
    (i)   Neutralising antibodies in plasma are particularly important where there is a blood-borne phase before the virus reaches its target tissue, e.g. poliomyelitis
    (ii)   Neutralising IgA antibodies in secretions from mucous membranes are important in preventing local infection, e.g. against influenzal attack on the respiratory mucosa
    (iii) Interferon
2. Cellular factors
    (i)   T-lymphocyte response and lymphokine stimulation of macrophages
    (ii)   Phagocytosis of virus by macrophages with subsequent interferon production, or transfer of the inducer to other interferon-producing cells

IMMUNITY TO PARASITIC INFECTION
1. *Protozoa*
Circulating antibody attacks the blood-borne stages but some protozoa such as malaria and trypanosomiasis undergo antigenic variation and may therefore avoid elimination.

2. *Helminths*
Immunity is associated with high levels of IgE (reaginic) antibodies. The local anaphylaxis provoked by exposure to antigen may prevent infestation by release of histamine or by egress of active antibodies and complement from the inflamed mucosa

OPPORTUNISTIC INFECTION

Opportunistic infections are usually found in patients whose body defences or immune reactivity are impaired. The infective agents may be recognised pathogens, or increasingly, may be organisms of low-pathogenicity often derived from the host flora.

Organisms of low pathogenicity or uncommon pathogens which are found in *opportunistic* infections include:

1. Fungi
   Candida albicans
   Cryptococcus neoformans
   Histoplasma capsulatum
   Aspergillus fumigatus
   Phycomycetes
   > *Mucor*
   > *Rhizopus*
   > *Absidia*

2. Bacteria
   Nocardia asteroides

3. Viruses
   Cytomegalovirus
   Varicella—herpes zoster ⎫
   Measles   ⎬ Disseminated infection
   Vaccinia   ⎭

Predisposing factors are:
1. *Disturbance of physical body defences*
   (i)   Surgery, e.g. infection by Bacteroides, Staphylococci
   (ii)   Trauma, e.g. Staphylococci
   (iii) Foreign-bodies including urinary and intravascular catheters—Gram-negative bacilli, fungi
   (iv)   Burns—Pseudomonas
2. *Alteration of flora* by antimicrobial drugs, especially of the mouth, intestine and skin—Candidiasis
3. *Immunosuppressive treatment*
   (i)   Corticosteroids ⎫
   (ii)   Irradiation   ⎬ various organisms, especially
   (iii) Chemotherapy   ⎭ Gram-negative bacilli

4. *Disorders of neutrophils* (see p. 18)
Staphylococci, Streptococci, Gram-negative bacilli, fungi

5. *Deficient humoral immunity,* as in chronic lymphatic leukaemia or multiple myeloma: Pyogenic cocci, Gram-negative bacilli, *Listeria monocytogenes, Pneumocystis carinii.*

6. *Deficient cellular immunity,* as in Hodgkin's disease: Fungi, viral infections especially cytomegalovirus, Brucella, *Cryptococcus neoformans.*

7. *Immunodeficiency of mixed type*—viral infections, *Pneumocystis carinii, Candida albicans.*

8. *Post-splenectomy—Streptococcus pneumoniae, Neisseria meningitidis, Haemophilus influenzae.*

FURTHER READING

Burnet, Sir F.M. & White, D.O. (1972) *Natural History of Infectious Disease,* 4th edn. London: Cambridge University Press.

Notkins, A.L. (1975) *Viral Immunology and Immunopathology.* London: Academic Press.

Rosen, P.R. (1976) Opportunistic fungal infections in patients with neoplastic disease. *Pathology Annual,* **11,** 255. New York: Appleton-Century-Crofts.

Strano, A.J. (1976) Light microscopy of selected viral diseases (morphology of viral inclusion bodies). *Pathology Annual,* **11,** 53. New York: Appleton-Century-Crofts.

Weinstein, L. & Swartz, M.N. (1974) *Pathologic Physiology,* ed. Sodeman, W.A. & Sodeman, W.A. p. 473. Philadelphia: Saunders.

Granulomatous diseases

TUBERCULOSIS

An infective condition caused by *Mycobacterium tuberculosis*.
Four 'strains' are of human importance:
1. Human
2. Bovine
3. Avian—a rare cause of human infection
4. Murine—has been used for immunisation purposes

Other potentially pathogenic mycobacteria are:
1. *M. balnei*
2. *M. ulcerans*   Skin infections
3. *M. kansasii*
4. *M. scrofulaceum*
5. *M. xenopei*
6. *M. intracellularis*

These are referred to as atypical, anonymous or opportunist
mycobacteria.

Routes of infection
1. Inhalation—pulmonary infection, the most common route
2. Ingestion—tonsillar or small intestinal infection (now
    uncommon as Bovine tuberculosis is eradicated)
3. Congenital (rare)
    (i)   Blood spread via the placenta
    (ii) Ingestion of infected amniotic fluid
4. Skin inoculation (very rare)

Primary infection
Initial infection leads in most cases to the formation of a
circumscribed cellular reaction (*the primary focus*) and lymphatic
spread of organisms to the regional lymph glands where a similar
response develops. The primary focus and the involved regional
glands are referred to as the *primary complex.*

In the majority of cases, infection is by inhalation and the primary
focus is usually found in a mid-zonal, sub-pleural situation (Ghon
focus) with associated involvement of hilar lymph glands.

The fully-developed lesion has a characteristic microscopic
appearance and is termed a *'tubercle'* or tuberculous follicle.

Development of the tubercle

The body's response to *M. tuberculosis* passes through the following stages:

1. A short-lived acute inflammatory response with exudation of polymorphs
2. Accumulation of macrophages forming a granuloma
3. Phagocytosis of tubercle bacilli followed by morphological changes in macrophages. The cells become eosinophilic, finely-granular, and their nuclei pale, oval or spindle-shaped. These altered macrophages supposedly resemble epithelial cells and are therefore termed *epithelioid cells*.
   They are poorly phagocytic (possibly related to loss of surface immunoglobulin receptors) but have a high secretory activity
4. Some macrophages fuse to form Langhan's giant cells characterised by a peripheral 'horse-shoe' arrangement of nuclei
5. Infiltration of surrounding tissue by specifically sensitised T-lymphocytes which secrete lymphokines including cytotoxic factors
6. Necrosis of the central zone with formation of structureless, finely-granular, eosinophilic material—*caseous necrosis*
7. Fibroblastic proliferation around the periphery with increasing collagenisation

The host response to tuberculosis

Resistance to tuberculosis varies between races and is modified by age, sex, hereditary and environmental factors.

Cell-mediated immunity is of far greater importance than humoral immunity in protection. The reactions of immunity include the development of delayed type hypersensitivity to tuberculoproteins derived from the bacillus, a form of bacterial allergy.

Immune responses

1. Macrophage phagocytosis and 'processing'
2. Accumulation of sensitised T-lymphocytes and lymphokine synthesis:
   (i) Mediators of acute inflammation, as seen at the site of tuberculin injection in a positive Mantoux test
   (ii) Macrophage chemotactic factor promotes monocyte emigration into the infected area
   (iii) Macrophage migration inhibition factor holds them in the area
   (iv) Macrophage activating factor and
   (v) Macrophage arming factor enhance the killing of Mycobacteria
   (vi) Cytotoxic factors which bring about destruction of macrophages and host tissue (caseous necrosis). Necrosis may be increased by ischaemia towards the centre of the tubercle
3. Fibroblastic proliferation (increased in immune patients?)

The course of the disease is dictated by:
1. Infecting dose
2. Virulence of the organism
3. Degree of resistance of the host

Effects of the primary complex
1. Systemic features
   In most cases there are no signs of ill-health; a few patients have:
   (i) Malaise
   (ii) Fever
   (iii) Erythema nodosum
   (iv) Raised ESR
   (v) Lymphocytosis
2. Local effects resulting from lymph gland enlargement
   (i) Peribronchial glands—lymph node compression syndrome
       a. Lung collapse
       b. Obstructive emphysema
       c. Bronchiectasis
   (ii) Cervical glands—disfiguring swelling in the neck

The fate of the primary complex
With most primary infections the development of specific cellular immunity is followed by progressive healing of the lesion.
1. Gradual destruction of bacilli (this may never be completed)
2. Progressive fibrosis and slow removal of caseous material
3. Calcification of persistent caseous debris or of the heavily collagenised scar tissue
Where the level of innate, and later specific, immunity is poor the lesion may spread directly, or through lymphatics, or through the blood stream.

Post-primary (adult or re-infection) tuberculosis

Pathogenesis
1. Re-infection by viable endogenous bacilli from a dormant primary lesion
2. Re-infection by exogenous bacilli in a patient rendered hypersensitive by previous infection but whose overall level of immunity is inadequate
Post-primary, like primary, infection is usually seen in the lung but the lesion is typically apical (Assmann Focus). There is early caseation and liquefaction because of previous sensitisation and the lesion may erode into a bronchus, discharge infected necrotic material, and produce a large cavity. Tuberculous bronchopneumonia may ensue, but progressive fibrocaseous destruction is more usual.

Spread of tuberculosis
1. Direct
   - (i) Lung
     - a. Acute tuberculous bronchopneumonia
     - b. Fibrocaseous pulmonary tuberculosis
     - c. Tuberculous empyema
   - (ii) Elsewhere
     Coalescence of caseous foci and liquefaction gives rise to a so-called 'cold-abscess'
2. Lymphatic spread to regional lymph glands is invariable in primary infection, uncommon in post-primary
3. Blood spread
   Organisms gain access to the circulation by:
   - (i) Lymphatic connections, e.g. thoracic duct
   - (ii) Rupture of a primary or post-primary focus into a vein
   - (iii) Erosion of a blood vessel in an involved lymph gland
   Two main patterns of blood spread are seen:
   - (i) Widespread dissemination—*miliary tuberculosis,* to liver, spleen, kidneys, lungs, bone-marrow, adrenals, prostate, seminal vesicles, endometrium, fallopian tubes and meninges
   - (ii) Single-organ involvement—implies that organisms carried to other sites are destroyed and infection progresses in an isolated organ. This may take many years to become clinically apparent by which time the pulmonary (or other) source of infection may have undergone healing by fibrosis and be difficult to identify. Common sites are meninges, kidneys, bone, fallopian tubes and epididymes
4. Infected sputum
   - (i) Tuberculous ulcers in the larynx
   - (ii) Ulcers in the small intestine (tuberculous enteritis)

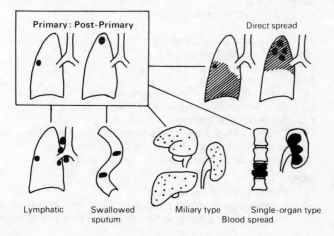

Spread of tuberculosis

Organ involvement in tuberculosis

1. Lungs
   (i) Primary (Ghon) focus
   (ii) Postprimary (Assmann) focus
   (iii) Tuberculous bronchopneumonia
   (iv) Fibrocaseous pulmonary tuberculosis
   (v) Cavitation (may become super-infected by moulds such as Aspergillus species)
   (vi) Miliary lesions
2. Alimentary tract
   (i) Primary focus (rare)
   (ii) Postprimary tuberculous enteritis
3. Central nervous system
   (i) Small cortical lesion (Rich's focus)
   (ii) Leptomeningitis arising from
       a. Direct haematogenous involvement of the choroid plexus
       b. Rupture of a Rich's focus
   Healed meningitis may give rise to hydrocephalus as a result of blockage of foramina by organised exudate.
   Pachymeningitis around the cord may arise by extension of vertebral infection.
   (iii) Ischaemic lesions resulting from endarteritis obliterans
   (iv) Tuberculous abscess (Tuberculoma) which may develop in areas of cortical ischaemic necrosis
4. Urinary system
   (i) Cortical lesions (appear first)
   (ii) Tubular spread to involve pyramids and calyces— tuberculous pyelonephritis
   (iii) Strictures at uretero-pelvic and uretero-vesical junctions
   (iv) Tuberculous 'pyonephrosis'
   (v) Spread to ureters, bladder, prostate and epididymis
5. Genital tract
   (i) Tuberculous salpingitis ⎫
   ⎬ result in infertility
   (ii) Tuberculous endometritis ⎭
   (iii) Tuberculous prostatitis
   (iv) Tuberculous epididymitis
6. Skeletal system
   (i) Early lesions near the epiphyseal line
   (ii) Destruction of cartilage and disc erosion
   (iii) Synovitis and arthritis
   (iv) Destruction of bone leads to pathological fractures and vertebral collapse (Pott's disease of the spine)
   (v) Spread along fascial planes (psoas abscess)
7. Skin
   (i) Primary lesion (very rare)
   (ii) Lupus vulgaris. Most common on the face and neck, and may result in extensive tissue destruction and scarring.

It is occasionally complicated by the development of squamous carcinoma

- (iii) Scrofuloderma. Involvement of the skin by direct extension from an underlying lymph gland
- (iv) Papulo-necrotic tuberculide—probably represents an extreme hypersensitivity reaction to infection elsewhere in the body
- (v) Erythema nodosum ⎫
                 ⎬ hypersensitivity reactions
- (vi) Erythema induratum ⎭

8. Serous cavities

   Tuberculosis of serous linings produces an exudative response characterised by an outpouring of protein-rich fluid containing large numbers of lymphocytes.
   - (i) Tuberculous pleurisy which may become an empyema
   - (ii) Tuberculous pericarditis may be followed by marked fibrosis and calcification producing constrictive pericarditis and cardiac failure
   - (iii) Tuberculous peritonitis may be a localised involvement associated with intestinal tuberculosis or salpingitis, or be generalised. This is a possible complication of laparotomy

9. Endocrine glands
   - (i) Tuberculosis of the adrenals (Addison's disease)
   - (ii) Tuberculous abscesses in the thyroid (rare)

10. Eyes
   - (i) Tubercles of the choroid in miliary spread
   - (ii) Phlyctenular conjunctivitis
   - (iii) Iridocyclitis

LEPROSY

A chronic inflammatory disease of low infectivity caused by *Mycobacterium leprae*.

Route of infection
1. By inhalation of droplet infection
2. Through intact skin by direct contact

When infection develops in the skin, the initial lesion is the *indeterminate macule*. Thereafter two major clinical forms may develop.

A. Lepromatous leprosy occurs in patients with low cell-mediated immunity to the organism which produces widespread infection.
1. Skin involvement
   - (i) Papules
   - (ii) Nodules covered by greasy skin
   - (iii) Diffuse thickening, e.g. leonine facies
   - (iv) Loss of hair

On histology the skin shows
   (i)   Dermal granulomata rich in histiocytes
   (ii)   Clear area between epidermis and affected dermis
   (iii) *Myco. leprae* in large numbers within histiocytes. These
        can be demonstrated using the Ziehl-Neelsen method
        without acid differentiation
   (iv) *Globi*—enlarged, fat-laden histiocytes containing
        clumped degenerate bacilli
  2. Nerve involvement
    (i)   Oedema and ischaemic necrosis
    (ii)   Progressive fibrosis
    (iii) Peripheral neuritis which is symmetrical
    (iv) Anaesthesia may lead to neuropathic arthropathy
         (Charcot's joints) and trophic ulcers
  3. Mucous membranes
    (i)   Nasal blockage and epistaxis
    (ii)   Ulceration of the nasal septum
    (iii) Ulceration and stenosis of the larynx
  4. Mouth—loss of upper incisors
  5. Eyes
    (i)   Punctate keratitis
    (ii)   Iritis
    (iii) Corneal ulceration
  6. Testes
    Testicular atrophy leading to sterility and gynaecomastia
  7. Death may result from
    (i)   Respiratory infection; pneumonia, tuberculosis
    (ii)   Septicaemia from chronic osteomyelitis following
        infection of bone marrow
    (iii) Renal failure due to chronic glomerulonephritis or
        amyloidosis

B. Tuberculoid leprosy develops when there is a high cell-mediated immunity and the infection is limited to skin and nerves.
  1. Skin lesions
    Scattered hypopigmented, anaesthetic areas showing
    anhidrosis
  2. Nerve involvement
    (i)   Destruction by granulomata
    (ii)   Repair by fibrosis with consequent thickening
    (iii) Anaesthesia, muscle wasting
    On histology these lesions show
    (i)   A mass of lymphocytes and epithelioid cells
    (ii)   Langhan's-type giant cells
    (iii) Very few organisms
    (iv) Skin involvement extending through the dermis and
        epidermis in continuity
    (v)   Caseous necrosis, sometimes within nerve lesions but
        not in the skin
Many of these features resemble those found in tuberculosis.

SARCOIDOSIS

This is a generalised disease of unknown aetiology characterised by widespread granuloma formation and protean clinical manifestations. It appears to be more common in communities which have recently eradicated tuberculosis and leprosy, but no definite link with these diseases has been established. Recent work suggests that sarcoidosis may result from simultaneous viral and mycobacterial infection in which case viral infection is responsible for the observed T-cell depression and mycobacteria exert a stimulant effect on B-lymphocyte function. Immune complexes may be formed which could be responsible for granuloma formation.

Immunological findings

1. Depressed T-cell function as shown by
   (i) Cutaneous anergy (as manifest by a negative Mantoux)
   (ii) Diminished response to non-specific mitogens
2. Exaggerated B-cell function as evidenced by increased circulating antibodies to a wide variety of antigens including EB virus, herpes simplex, rubella, measles, and parainfluenzae

The sarcoid granuloma consists of:

1. A well circumscribed collection of epithelioid macrophages
2. Giant-cells, mainly Langhan's but also of foreign-body type
3. Inclusion bodies found in giant-cells (and occasionally in epithelioid cells)
   (i) Residual bodies about 1μm in diameter which are end-stage phagosomes
   (ii) Schaumann bodies—laminated, basophilic conchoidal bodies which when large become extracellular
   (iii) Asteroid bodies—small star-shaped refractile inclusions
4. An outer narrow zone of lymphocytes
5. A collar of fibrous tissue
6. Central necrosis is uncommon and mild in degree. The reticulin framework is preserved whereas in caseation it is usually destroyed

These appearances although suggestive of sarcoidosis are not specific and may be found in many other conditions.

Sarcoid-like granulomata may be found in:

1. Bacterial diseases
   (i) Non-caseating tuberculosis
   (ii) Brucellosis
   (iii) Leprosy
   (iv) Mesenteric adenitis due to *Yersinia enterocolitica*
2. Virus diseases
   (i) Cat scratch disease
   (ii) *Lymphogranuloma venereum*
3. Fungal diseases
   (i) Histoplasmosis
   (ii) Coccidioidomycosis
   (iii) Blastomycosis

4. Protozoal diseases
    (i)   Leishmaniasis
    (ii) Toxoplasmosis
5. Foreign-body/Mineral granulomata
    (i)   Corn-starch grains (used in surgical glove powder)
    (ii) Talc
    (iii) Silica
    (iv) Beryllium (used in fluorescent tubes)
    (v)   Zirconium (used in deodorants)
6. Hypersensitivity reactions
    (i)   Allergic alveolitis
    (ii) Arteritis
7. Hodgkin's disease in tissues not directly involved by neoplasm
   (e.g. liver/spleen)
8. Crohn's disease
9. Primary biliary cirrhosis
10. 'Local' sarcoid reactions in lymph glands
    (i)   Draining a wide variety of tumours
    (ii) In association with chronic cholecystitis
          (Cholegranulomatous lymphadenitis)

Organ involvement in sarcoidosis
1. *Lungs*
    (i)   Widespread 'miliary' lesions
    (ii) Linear fibrosis radiating from the hilum
    (iii) Diffuse fibrosis which may progress to 'honeycomb lung'
    (iv) Collapse secondary to bronchial obstruction (rare)
2. *Lymph glands* Hilar gland involvement is common
3. *Skin*
    (i)   Erythema nodosum is common
    (ii) Boeck's sarcoid—purple/red papules, nodules or plaques
          found principally on the face, as well as on the extensor
          surfaces of the arms and upper back
    (iii) Darier-Roussy sarcoid—where the lesions are
          subcutaneous rather than intracutaneous and are found
          on the trunk
    (iv) Lupus pernio—characterised by indurated, erythematous
          bluish-red macules and plaques found on the face, ears
          and fingers
4. *Eyes*
    (i)   Uveitis—inflammation of the iris and ciliary body
    (ii) Conjunctivitis
    (iii) Retinal lesions
    (iv) Keratoconjunctivitis sicca
5. *Salivary glands* resulting in enlargement and loss of secretion.
Sarcoidosis is one of the many causes of Mikulicz's syndrome
(bilateral enlargement and loss of secretion in salivary and
lachrymal glands). Involvement is sometimes accompanied by
uveitis and pyrexia—uveoparotid fever (Heerfordt's syndrome).

6. *Liver* involvement, whilst common, is rarely of clinical significance.

7. *Spleen.* Sarcoidosis is a rare cause of mild to moderate splenomegaly

8. *Bone.* Small cystic lesions in the phalanges of the feet and hands

9. *Heart.* Myocardial granulomata and fibre atrophy may lead to heart failure or conduction defects

10. *Pituitary and hypothalamus.* Sarcoidosis is a rare cause of diabetes insipidus

11. *Central nervous system* (uncommon)
    - (i) Meningoencephalitis
    - (ii) Peripheral neuropathy
    - (iii) Transverse myelitis

12. *Kidneys* mainly involved by nephrocalcinosis consequent upon hypercalcaemia and hypercalciuria which result from vitamin D sensitivity with increased uptake of calcium from the gut.

13. *Skeletal muscle*—sarcoid myopathy.

Histological diagnosis
1. Kveim test. This consists of an intradermal injection of a saline suspension of a sarcoid lymph gland or spleen. A positive reaction, which takes about 6 weeks to develop, appears as a firm nodule with the features of a sarcoid granuloma on histology
2. Biopsy of lymph gland, liver, skeletal muscle, labial salivary glands, skin or even lung.

SYPHILIS
Syphilis is one of a group of diseases spread principally by sexual contact—venereal diseases. The group comprises
1. Syphilis—infection by *Treponema pallidum*
2. Gonorrhoea—*Neisseria gonorrhoeae*
3. Lymphogranuloma venereum—Chlamydia/Bedsonia
4. Chancroid (soft sore)—*Haemophilus ducreyi*
5. Donovanosis—*Donovania granulomatis*
6. Reiters syndrome—aetiology unknown
    - (i) Urethritis
    - (ii) Conjunctivitis
    - (iii) Arthritis
7. Non-specific urethritis—aetiology unknown

Syphilis can be congenital, resulting from trans-placental infection, or acquired.

Natural history of acquired syphilis

1. Inoculation followed by an incubation period of 2–4 weeks but possibly 10–90 days
2. The *primary lesion* which is usually present for 6–8 weeks
3. Involvement of regional lymph glands and spread into the blood stream
4. The *secondary stage* may take up to 9 months to disappear
5. The *latent stage* where there are no signs and symptoms but the infection is still present and active
6. The *tertiary stage* becomes clinically apparent 3–10 years after infection
7. Later involvement of the cardiovascular and nervous systems. This may take up to 20–40 years to present clinically. The late nervous system involvement is sometimes referred to as quaternary syphilis

Primary syphilis

The primary lesion is the chancre, which when fully developed is a hard, painless, indurated ulcer with regular, well-demarcated margins. Histologically there is:

1. Ulceration
2. Underlying granulation tissue
3. Endothelial proliferation in small blood vessels
4. Heavy plasma-cell and lymphocytic infiltration
5. Healing by fibrosis producing a small scar
   Spirochaetes may be demonstrable by a silver impregnation method such as the Levaditi stain

Secondary syphilis

The lesions are very variable:

1. Skin rashes (syphilides)
   (i) Macular
   (ii) Papular, which in warm and moist parts of the body may produce large fleshy masses—condylomata lata
   (iii) Pustular destructive lesions (rare)
2. Mucous membranes
   (i) Mucous patch—a grey white membrane with a dull-red margin found in the mouth, pharynx and larynx
   (ii) 'Snail-track' ulcers
3. Lymphadenitis
4. Hepatitis
5. Iritis
6. Arthritis, bursitis and periostitis
7. Meningitis (rare)

Tertiary syphilis

The characteristic lesion is the *gumma*. This comprises:

1. A central zone of structured necrosis in which the original architecture can usually be distinguished
2. A surrounding zone of epithelioid cells and occasional giant cells.
3. Granulation tissue heavily infiltrated by plasma cells and lymphocytes
4. Fibrosis
5. Endarteritis obliterans

Lesions are found in:

1. Skin and subcutaneous tissue
   (i) Nodular skin lesions
   (ii) Subcutaneous gummata which ulcerate and heal slowly with thin, poorly-formed scars
2. Mucous membranes
   (i) Localised gummata in mouth, pharynx, larynx and nasal septum
   (ii) Diffuse involvement of the tongue with leucoplakia
   These lesions are very prone to malignant change
3. Bones
   Lesions commence in the periosteum and provoke new bone formation but later spread into cortical bone and have a destructive effect ('worm-eaten' skull)
4. Liver
   Gummata followed by irregular fibrosis break the liver up into distorted lobes—'hepar lobatum'
5. Testis
6. Rare sites—muscles and joints, gastrointestinal tract, lung, spleen, urinary tract

Cardiovascular syphilis (tertiary)

1. Heart
   Gumma (very rare). The diagnosis may be suggested by the finding of bundle-branch block
2. Small arteries
   (i) Intimal proliferation
   (ii) Adventitial fibrosis
   produce endarteritis obliterans which may lead to ischaemic damage

3. Aorta—syphilitic mesaortitis
    This is the commonest manifestation of tertiary syphilis and
    is an important cause of death
    Pathogenesis
    (i)   Infection around adventitial vessels spreads into the wall
          along vasa vasorum
    (ii) Endarteritis obliterans develops in these small nutrient
          vessels
    (iii) Ischaemia leads to necrosis of the media with
          destruction of elastic lamina
    These changes are most marked in the proximal part of the
    thoracic aorta
    Effects
    (i)   Aneurysm formation
    (ii) Aortic incompetence
    (iii) Coronary ostial stenosis leading to myocardial ischaemia

Neurosyphilis (? quaternary)
Treponema invade the CNS in up to 20% of cases during the early
stages of syphilitic infection. In the absence of treatment
approximately half of these patients will develop signs of
neurosyphilis after a lapse of many years.
1. Connective tissues and blood vessels (meningovascular)
    (i)   Leptomeningitis which may be complicated by cranial
          nerve palsies and internal hydrocephalus
    (ii) Pachymeningitis
    (iii) Gummata in the meninges
    (iv) Endarteritis obliterans leading to cerebral infarcts
2. Parenchymal involvement
    (i)   General paralysis of the insane (G.P.I.)
          A chronic syphilitic encephalitis with widespread lesions
          and diverse motor, sensory, and psychiatric symptoms
          The main *pathological features* are:
          a. Degeneration of nerve cells and fibres with cerebral
             atrophy
          b. Proliferation and hyperplasia of microglia forming
             'rod-cells'
          c. Reactive proliferation of astrocytes—gliosis
          d. Thickening of leptomeninges
          e. Perivascular infiltration by lymphocytes and plasma
             cells
    (ii) Tabes dorsalis
          This is the equivalent lesion in the spinal cord and
          involves lower sensory neurones.
          Pathological features:
          a. Wasting of the posterior roots
          b. Thickening of the pia-arachnoid
          c. Gross demyelination of the dorsal columns
          Effects:
          a. Loss of coordination with ataxia
          b. Deep anaesthesia resulting in Charcot's joints and
             penetrating ulcers

Congenital syphilis

The fetus may be overwhelmed by infection and die. In those that survive, the lesions found during the first 2 years are similar to those of the secondary stage. Many of the lesions appearing in the third year and after are of the gummatous type. The scars or deformities resulting from early or late lesions which have healed are termed *stigmata.*

A. *Early lesions*
1. Bullous rash
2. Mucous patches—syphilitic rhinitis
3. Liver—diffuse pericellular fibrosis ('cirrhosis')
4. Lungs—pale consolidation seen in some fatal cases
5. Bones—osteochondritis
6. Eyes—choroiditis

B. *Late lesions*
1. Eyes—interstitial keratitis
2. Neurosyphilis
3. Bones—gummatous periostitis most commonly seen in the tibia (sabre tibia)
4. Deafness

C. *Stigmata*
1. Facial disfigurement
    (i) Saddle nose
    (ii) 'Bossing' of frontal bones
    (iii) High arched palate
2. Teeth
    (i) Hutchinson's teeth, notching of the permanent incisors resulting from suppression of the middle of the three denticles from which the tooth develops
    (ii) Moon's molars—underdeveloped first lower molars
3. Rhagades—healed radiating fissures around the corners of the mouth
4. Perforation of palate or nasal septum (gummatous)
5. Optic atrophy

FURTHER READING

Mitchell, D.N. Scadding, J.G., Heard, B.E. & Hinson, K.F.W. (1977) Sarcoidosis: histopathological definition and clinical diagnosis. *Journal of Clinical Pathology,* **30,** 395.

Rees, R.J.W. & Ridley, D.S. (1973) Bacteriology and pathology of leprosy. *Recent Advances in Clinical Pathology,* 6. ed. Dyke, S.C. Edinburgh: Churchill Livingstone.

Seal, R.M.E. (1971) The pathology of tuberculosis. *British Journal of Hospital Medicine,* **5,** 783.

Hypertension

CONTROL OF BLOOD PRESSURE
The general level of the systemic arterial blood pressure is maintained by three mechanisms:
1. Catecholamine production
2. Renin-angiotensin system
3. Aldosterone production—sodium retention

Regulation of the blood pressure against this background of endocrine control is achieved by the baro-receptor mechanism and autonomic nervous system.

1. Catecholamine production
Catecholamines are produced principally by the chromaffin cells of the adrenal medulla.
Adrenaline increases:
- (i) Heart rate
- (ii) Cardiac output
- (iii) Systolic blood pressure

Noradrenaline increases:
- (i) Peripheral resistance
- (ii) Both systolic and diastolic pressure

2. Renin-angiotensin system
Renin is an enzyme produced by the juxta-glomerular apparatus (JGA) in the kidney. It acts on a substrate (angiotensinogen) found in the α-2 globulin fraction of plasma to form a decapeptide angiotensin II.
Release of renin is stimulated by:
- (i) Reduction in renal perfusion pressure
- (ii) Hyponatraemia
- (iii) ß-adrenergic stimulation

Angiotensin II has the following effects:
- (i) Stimulates aldosterone secretion
- (ii) Increases blood pressure
- (iii) Modifies the excretion of water and electrolytes by a direct action on the kidney
- (iv) Stimulates thirst by an action on the central nervous system

3. Aldosterone production—sodium retention
Aldosterone is produced by the zona glomerulosa cells of the adrenal cortex, its main actions are:
- (i) Increases potassium excretion
- (ii) Increases sodium reabsorption, mainly in the distal tubules
- (iii) Produces a metabolic alkalosis by interfering with urinary acidification

Excessive production of aldosterone leads to hypokalaemia and hypernatraemia, with an associated moderate rise in blood pressure.

Excessive production can be either primary, or secondary to an increase in renin/angiotensin formation.

Causes

(i)   Primary aldosteronism
   a. Adrenocortical adenoma with suppression of renin and angiotensin as a consequence of sodium retention (Conn's syndrome)
   b. Adrenocortical micronodular hyperplasia
   c. Aldosterone-secreting carcinoma of the adrenal or ovary (very rare)

(ii) Secondary aldosteronism
   a. Diuretic therapy with increased Na^+ loss
   b. Na^+ losing renal disease, e.g. chronic pyelonephritis
   c. Cardiac failure
   d. Cirrhosis of the liver
   e. Nephrotic syndrome
   f. Malignant hypertension
   g. 'Toxaemia' of pregnancy
   h. Combination-type contraceptive pill
   i. Renal artery stenosis
   j. Renin-secreting tumours of the kidney
   k. Bartter's syndrome (hypertrophy of the JGA)

4. Autonomic nervous system

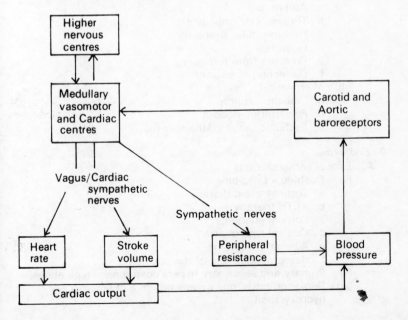

CLASSIFICATION AND CAUSES OF SYSTEMIC HYPERTENSION

Investigation of the majority of patients with hypertension (BP>160/95 mm Hg) reveals no underlying primary disease and the condition is termed *essential* hypertension.

It has been proposed that essential hypertension is an exaggeration of the tendency for blood pressure to rise with age, and that it results from a repeated sequence in which autonomic nervous overactivity results in a small rise in blood pressure and produces changes in the kidney which maintain the raised level and becomes the basis for a further incremental rise.

In about 15% of patients an underlying cause is found and these cases are termed *secondary*. When the diastolic pressure is in excess of 120 mm Hg and there is papilloedema, the hypertension may be designated *'malignant'* in type as it carries a poor prognosis. The malignant phase of hypertension is associated with characteristic pathological features.

Possible causes of *secondary* hypertension are:

1. *Renal diseases*
   - (i)   Parenchymal
     - a. Chronic pyelonephritis
     - b. Acute or chronic glomerulonephritis
     - c. Polycystic disease
     - d. Amyloidosis
     - e. Tumours
     - f. Hydronephrosis
   - (ii) Renal artery stenosis/obstruction
     - a. Atheroma
     - b. Thrombosis/embolism
     - c. Fibromuscular dysplasia
     - d. Ligatures
     - e. Pressure from tumours
     - f. Dissecting aneurysm
   - (iii) Microvascular disease
     - a. Diabetic nephropathy
     - b. Polyarteritis nodosa
     - c. Systemic lupus erythematosus

2. *Endocrine*
   - A. Excess corticosteroids
     - (i)   Cushing's syndrome
       - a. Corticosteroid therapy
       - b. ACTH therapy
       - c. Cortical adenoma
       - d. Cortical hyperplasia
       - e. Adrenal carcinoma
       - f. Basophil adenoma of the pituitary
     - (ii) Primary and secondary hyperaldosteronism (see above)
     - (iii) Deoxycorticosterone excess due to a defect in 17-hydroxylation

(iv)   Adrenogenital syndrome resulting from absence of 11-ß-hydroxylase. This leads to excessive production of 11-deoxycorticosterone and 11-deoxycortisol which exert mineralocorticoid effects (see p. 104)

B.   Excess catecholamines
(i)   Phaeochromocytoma—a tumour of chromaffin cells. 90% are found in the adrenal medulla: rare sites include sympathetic ganglia around the aorta and inferior vena cava and in the wall of the bladder. These tumours secrete large quantities of noradrenaline/adrenaline
(ii)   Treatment with indirect sympathomimetics (amphetamine, tyramine) in combination with monoamine oxidase inhibitors

C.   Pituitary causes
(i)   Acidophil adenoma giving rise to acromegaly
(ii)   Basophil adenoma with excessive ACTH production

D.   Renin-producing tumours of the kidney (very rare)

3. *Cardiovascular causes*
(i)   Coarctation of the aorta
(ii)   High cardiac output states produce a rise in blood pressure but do not result in the systemic pathological lesions of hypertension (see p. 91)

4. *Neurological causes* (usually giving a transient or terminal elevation)
(i)   Raised intracranial pressure
a.   Trauma
b.   Tumour
c.   Abscess
d.   Haemorrhage
(ii)   Lesions of hypothalamus and brain-stem
(iii)   Psychogenic—anxiety state

PATHOLOGICAL EFFECTS OF 'BENIGN' HYPERTENSION

1. *Blood vessels*
A.   Arterioles
(i)   Hyalinisation; this is seen in ageing but is accentuated by hypertension. It consists of the accumulation of homogeneous eosinophilic material initially under the endothelium but later replacing the entire wall and occurs in many organs. It is seen most frequently in the kidney (afferent arterioles) spleen, pancreas, and adrenals. The hyaline deposit contains some fibrin, glycoprotein, lipid and cholesterol and is presumed to originate from the plasma

B. Small and medium-sized arteries
    (i)   Medial muscular hypertrophy and later fibrosis
    (ii)   Duplication of the elastic lamina
    (iii) Intimal proliferation
    (iv)   Micro-aneurysm formation in the small perforating
           arteries (less than 1 mm diameter) of the brain,
           especially in the basal ganglia and subcortical areas.
           Such aneurysms are found with increasing age, but they
           are found earlier and in greater numbers in hypertensive
           patients. There is loss of the muscular media and the
           wall consists of dilated intima and adventitia. Some
           micro-aneurysms contain subintimal hyaline deposits
           which stain for fibrin and fat (lipohyalinosis) and these
           lesions are particularly prone to rupture
C. Large arteries
    Increase in severity of atherosclerosis and its results

2. *Kidneys* (hypertensive nephrosclerosis)
   A. Gross appearances
       (i)   Normal or reduced size
       (ii)   Granular surface
   B. Glomeruli
       (i)   Thickening of basement membrane
       (ii)   Loss of cellularity
       (iii) Hyalinisation
   C. Bowman's capsule
       (i)   Deposition of collagen on inside of capsule
       (ii)   Less frequently, dilatation of Bowman's space and
              collapse of the glomerulus
   D. Tubules
       Variable atrophy, with occasional casts.
   Most of these changes probably result from ischaemia

3. *Heart*
       (i)   Left ventricular hypertrophy
       (ii)   Increased coronary atherosclerosis
       (iii) Focal myocardial fibrosis

4. *Brain*
       (i)   Massive intra-cerebral haemorrhage
       (ii)   Perivascular ischaemic atrophy maximal in the globus
              pallidus
       (iii) Multiple small infarcts
       (iv)   Multiple small haemorrhages
       (v)   Microaneurysms

PATHOLOGICAL EFFECTS OF MALIGNANT HYPERTENSI

1. *Blood vessels*
    A. Arterioles
       Fibrinoid 'necrosis' of the arteriolar wall in which pyknotic
       nuclear fragments and red blood cells may be seen. Found in
       the kidney, pancreas, adrenal, mesentery, brain, eye, heart
       and liver. Such arteriolar necrosis is also a feature of:
       (i)   Systemic lupus erythematosus
       (ii) Polyarteritis nodosa
       (iii) Haemolytic-uraemic syndrome
       (iv) Irradiation
    B. Arteries
       Endarteritis fibrosa: Concentric lamellar connective tissue and
       mucinous thickening of the intima ('onion-skin' thickening)
       which narrows the lumen. Also seen in:
       (i)   Progressive systemic sclerosis
       (ii) Post-partum acute renal failure
       (iii) Haemolytic-uraemic syndrome
       (iv) Rejection after transplantation

2. *Kidney*
    A. Gross appearances
       (i)   Size is variable
       (ii) Smooth surface
       (iii) Subcapsular petechial haemorrhages
    B. Glomeruli
       (i)   Patchy fibrinoid necrosis of tufts
       (ii) Occasionally complete infarction of tufts
    C. Bowman's capsule
       (i)   Deposition of fibrin in the capsular space
       (ii) Occasional epithelial 'crescent' formation

3. *Brain* (hypertensive vascular crisis)
    A. Gross appearances
       (i)   Oedema
       (ii) Petechial haemorrhages
    B. Microscopic appearances
       (i)   Fibrinoid necrosis of arterioles and small arteries
       (ii) Perivascular cuffing by lymphocytes

PULMONARY HYPERTENSION
The normal pressure in the pulmonary artery is about
20/10 mm Hg. Pulmonary hypertension is characterised by
pressures in excess of 30/15 mm Hg.

Causes of pulmonary arterial hypertension
1. Increased pulmonary venous pressure
    (i)   Chronic left ventricular failure
    (ii) Mitral stenosis
    Rare causes:
    (iii) Left atrial myxoma
    (iv) Cor triatriatum
    (v)   Idiopathic thrombosis of pulmonary veins
    (vi) Compression of veins by mediastinal neoplasm
    (vii) Veno-occlusive disease
2. Increased pulmonary vascular resistance
    (i)   Obstruction to pulmonary arteries/arterioles
        a. Recurrent thromboemboli (obliterative pulmonary
           hypertension)
        b. *In situ* thrombosis
        c. Tumour fragments
        d. Ova of Schistosoma mansoni
    (ii) Destruction of pulmonary vasculature
        a. Severe pulmonary fibrosis, as in tuberculosis,
           silicosis, etc.
        b. Bronchiectasis
        c. Emphysema and chronic bronchitis
    (iii) Destruction associated with alveolar-capillary diffusion
          block
        a. Pneumokonioses
        b. Sarcoidosis
        c. Progressive systemic sclerosis
        d. Fibrosing alveolitis
    (iv) Vasoconstriction due to hypoxia
        a. Emphysema and chronic bronchitis
        b. High altitude
        c. Pulmonary oedema
        d. Primary pulmonary hypertension
        e. Pickwickian syndrome—extreme obesity, somnolence,
           hypercapnia, hypoxia and polycythaemia
3. Increased pulmonary blood-flow resulting from left to right
   shunts
    (i)   Atrial septal defect
    (ii) Persistent ductus arteriosus
    (iii) Ventricular septal defect
    (iv) Anomalous pulmonary venous drainage into the right
          atrium or superior vena cava
    (v)   Persistent truncus arteriosus
    (vi) Cor triloculare

Blood vessels of the lung
1. Bronchial arteries—thick walled, muscular, systemic pressure.
2. Elastic pulmonary arteries ($>1000\mu$ m diameter)
   (i) Fetus and up to 6 months old—thick walled, elastic fibres are long, non-branched and parallel
   (ii) After infancy—thin walled, elastic fibres are branched, fragmented and form a loose network
3. Muscular pulmonary arteries (100 – 1000μm diameter)
4. Pulmonary arterioles ($<100\mu$m diameter)
5. Pulmonary capillaries
6. Pulmonary venules (identical appearance to arterioles)
7. Pulmonary veins

Changes in the pulmonary vasculature in hypertension
1. Elastic arteries
   (i) Where hypertension has been present from birth there is persistence of the fetal elastic pattern
   (ii) Medial hypertrophy
   (iii) Mucoid degeneration
   (iv) Atherosclerosis
   (v) Intimal fibrosis, dilation, and thinning of the media (late feature)
2. Muscular arteries
   (i) Medial hypertrophy with intimal proliferation
   (ii) Progressive fibro-elastic occlusion
   (iii) Localised dilatations
   (iv) Rupture of dilatations giving rise to haemosiderosis
   (v) Necrotising arteritis (rare)

Effects of pulmonary hypertension
Right ventricular hypertrophy (= Cor pulmonale, where the cause is a primary lung disease) and failure (see p. 90)

FURTHER READING
Gray, I.R. (1972) Control of blood pressure. *British Medical Journal,* **2**, 31.
Robertson, J.S. (1974) Endocrine aspects of hypertension. *British Journal of Hospital Medicine,* **11**, 707.
Tarazi, R.C. & Gifford, R.W. (1974) Systemic arterial pressure. In *Pathologic Physiology,* 5th edn., ed. Sodeman, W.A. & Sodeman, W.A. p. 177. Philadelphia: Saunders.

Atherosclerosis and aneurysms

Atherosclerosis is a disease which affects the intima of arteries. It appears as focal thickenings or plaques composed of fibrous tissue and lipid deposits. Atherosclerosis is not synonymous with arteriosclerosis. This term includes a number of diseases characterised by thickening of arterial vessels:

Classification of arteriosclerosis
- (i) Intimal thickening with lipid deposition—atherosclerosis
- (ii) Hyaline thickening
- (iii) Medial fibrosis } ageing, diabetes and hypertension
- (iv) Fibrous intimal proliferation (arteriosclerosis obliterans)
- (v) Medial hypertrophy } Hypertension
- (vi) Medial calcification—Monckeberg's sclerosis

PATHOLOGY OF ATHEROSCLEROSIS
This disease is generally considered to pass through three stages, the fatty streak, the fibro-fatty plaque, and the complicated lesion.

1. *Fatty streaks* in the aortic intima can be found even in the first two decades of life, especially in the aortic valve region, around the ductus scar, and just below the intercostal ostia. Some of the lipid is found in endothelial cells overlying the streaks, but the majority is found within 'foam-cells' in the intima. These foam-cells arise from two sources: the majority are lipid-containing smooth muscle cells—'myogenic' foam-cells, and a small proportion are macrophages probably derived from circulating monocytes. Most of the lipid in these lesions is intracellular and can therefore be mobilised and resorbed under certain circumstances, e.g. a low-lipid diet.

2. *Fibro-fatty plaques* represent the typical lesions seen in middle and old age. They consist of lipid accumulations, fibro-elastic tissue, and proliferated smooth-muscle cells in the intima. Earlier lesions contain myogenic foam-cells and a few macrophages in the subendothelial region, but in the later stages the lipid is predominantly extracellular and is found as free fat or cholesterol crystals in a central mass of necrotic material. New vessels develop from the vasa vasorum and adventitia and infiltrate the base of the plaque.

3. *Complicated lesions.* The fibro-fatty plaques can be complicated by:
- (i) Superimposed thrombosis

74

(ii)   Haemorrhage into the plaque from the vasa vasorum
(iii) Rupture and ulceration with discharge of necrotic debris
(iv)   Calcification

In order to understand the various theories of pathogenesis, the normal structure and the physiological pressure effects acting on large arteries must be understood.

1. Structure of a large artery

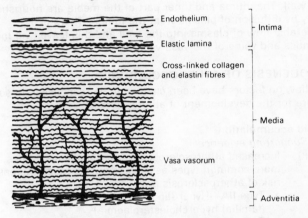

(i)   *Endothelium* has a structure similar to that found in capillaries and is freely permeable to fluid and electrolytes. It also allows slow leakage of large molecules, e.g. protein and lipoproteins, from the plasma into the intima

(ii) *Intima* is the loose fibro-elastic tissue lying between the endothelium and internal elastic lamina. It becomes thicker with age and shows a gradual increase in its content of smooth muscle cells

(iii) *The media* is composed of collagen fibres, elastic tissue and smooth muscle cells. Its main function is to resist the expansive force of the blood pressure, and convert a pulsatile into a continuous flow.

(iv) The outermost layer consists of loose fibrocellular tissue—*the adventitia*. It contains nerve fibres, lymphatics and small nutrient arteries associated with the vessel wall.

(v)   *Ground substance* fills the interstices of the wall and is most abundant in the intima. It binds or retards larger molecules passing through the wall, thus acting as a fine-pored filter, and is composed predominantly of acid mucopolysaccharides (glycosaminoglycans) and glycoproteins

(vi) *The vasa vasorum* are the small blood vessels which enter from the adventitia and supply the outer 2/3 of the wall

2. Pressure effects on the wall

Arterial walls are subjected to a considerable compressive force amounting, for example, to about 50 kg/cm² in the aorta. This compressive force is gradually converted into a tangential force by the elastic laminae and muscle fibres of the media. The vasa vasorum can only nourish those parts of the wall where the intramural compressive force is equal to or less than the capillary blood pressure, and such conditions are found only in the outer 2/3 of the wall. The intima and inner part of the media are nourished entirely by diffusion of plasma from the lumen. There is a considerable flow of plasma into the wall and this leaves via the lymphatics and veins of the vasa vasorum.

PATHOGENESIS OF ATHEROSCLEROSIS

The following factors have been claimed to be responsible in some measure for the development of atherosclerosis.

A. Lipid accumulation

1. *Supporting evidence*
    (i)   Increased atherosclerosis in hyperlipidaemic states. The more common types associated with a much increased risk of atherosclerosis are:
        a. Type IIA—Hyperß lipoproteinaemia (familial hypercholesterolaemia)
        b. Type IIB—Overindulgence hyperlipidaemia
        c. Type IV—Endogenous hypertriglyceridaemia (raised pre-ß-lipoprotein)
    (ii) Increased atherosclerosis in hypercholesterolaemia resulting from primary (familial) or secondary deficiency of Lecithin-Cholesterol Acyltransferase (LCAT)
    (iii) Production of fatty plaques in experimental animals by feeding with a high cholesterol diet
    (iv) Analysis of atheromatous plaques reveals 10 or more times the normal lipid content of the intima. The increase is predominantly made up of low-density lipoproteins
    (v)   High α-lipoprotein levels protect against coronary atherosclerosis probably by aiding the removal of cholesterol deposited in the intima by the ß- and pre-ß-lipoproteins
2. *Possible mechanisms*
    (i)   Excess low density lipoproteins in the plasma
    (ii) Retention of lipoproteins passing through the wall by changes in the filtration characteristics of the ground substance
    (iii) Altered permeability of the endothelium possibly initiated by platelet aggregation, allowing more plasma lipids to enter the wall. This could result in intimal oedema and trapping of lipoproteins

    (iv) Defective metabolism of the smooth muscle cells with a relative lack of hydrolytic enzymes leading to saturation of the lysosomal lipoprotein disposal system

    (v) Leakage from newly-formed vasa vasorum in fibro-fatty plaques

3. *Effects*

    (i) Alteration in the ground substance

    (ii) Proliferation of smooth muscle cells—frequently monoclonal

    (iii) Accumulation of 'foam' cells

    (iv) Increase in connective tissue fibres

    (v) Necrosis and inflammation in advanced lesions (necrogenic effect of lipids)

B. Haemodynamic stress

1. *Supporting evidence*

    (i) Increased severity in large vessels where the tangential shearing forces are greatest

    (ii) Association with systemic hypertension

    (iii) Absence from veins, and minimal involvement of the pulmonary circulation (except in pulmonary hypertension)

    (iv) More frequently found at sites of branching

2. *Effects of stress*

    (i) Endothelial desquamation and platelet adherence

    (ii) Polymerisation of the ground substance which alters its filtration properties

    (iii) Formation of new collagen and elastin fibres

    (iv) Intimal thickening resulting from connective tissue and smooth muscle cell proliferation

    (v) Rupture of the internal elastic lamina

C. Organisation of surface thrombosis

Supporting evidence

    (i) Microscopic appearances of organised mural thrombus may be identical to those of an atheromatous plaque

    (ii) Deposition of fibrin and platelets on vascular endothelium is a frequent event

    (iii) Atheromatous plaques contain large quantities of fibrinogen and fibrin

    (iv) Hyperlipidaemic states are also associated with a decreased clotting time and impaired fibrinolysis

Multifactorial causation

The currently held view is that surface thrombosis may follow the earliest changes of atherosclerosis where there is already some damage to the endothelium, but that it does not initiate the disease Likewise, raised circulating lipids increase the severity of atherosclerosis but their accumulation is probably secondary to an initiating factor such as mechanical stress, altered endothelial permeability, or defective metabolism of the arterial wall.

EFFECTS OF ATHEROSCLEROSIS
1. Progressive occlusion leading to ischaemia
2. Superimposed thrombosis with sudden occlusion producing infarction
3. Haemorrhage into a plaque
4. Rupture of a plaque leading to embolism
5. Aneurysm formation

ANEURYSMS
An aneurysm is a localised dilatation of an artery or part of the heart consequent upon weakening of its wall.

1. *Large and medium-sized arteries.* Aneurysms may result from:
   (i) Atherosclerosis. This is the commonest cause. Secondary weakening of the media gives rise to fusiform or saccular dilatations usually in the abdominal portion of the aorta
   (ii) Syphilis. The mesaortitis of tertiary syphilis can lead to aneurysms in the thoracic aorta
   (iii) Cystic medionecrosis. In this disorder there is focal loss of elastin and accumulation of acid mucopolysaccharide in the media with subsequent cystic degeneration and splitting of the vessel giving rise to a 'dissecting aneurysm'
   (iv) Trauma, especially in arteries of the legs
   (v) Congenital defects. A congenital deficiency of the media and elastica in cerebral arteries leads to 'berry' aneurysm formation
   (iv) Polyarteritis nodosa
   (vii) Infection of the vessel wall by bacteria brought there by infected emboli giving rise to 'mycotic' aneurysms, e.g. in bacterial endocarditis

2. *Small arteries.* Microscopic dilatations of small arteries (microaneurysms) which predispose to rupture are found in:
   (i) Systemic hypertension, in small intracerebral arteries
   (ii) Pulmonary hypertension, as dilatation lesions in muscular arteries
   (iii) Diabetic retinopathy

FURTHER READING
American Journal of Pathology (1977) Symposium on atherosclerosis—a new look at the problem. *American Journal of Pathology*, **86**, 656.

Porter, R. & Knight, J. (Eds.) (1973) Atherogenesis: initiating factors. Ciba Foundation Symposium, 12. Associated Scientific Publishers.

Thrombosis and embolism

Thrombosis is the formation of a solid mass from the constituents of the circulating blood within the vascular system. The solid (or semi-solid) mass is called a *thrombus*.

CAUSES OF THROMBOSIS

These are best considered under the three headings originally proposed by Virchow in 1856:

A. Changes in the vessel wall
B. Changes in blood flow
C. Changes in the constitution of the blood

A. Changes in the vessel wall

1. Arteries
   - (i) Atherosclerosis
   - (ii) Inflammation
       - a. Direct involvement in wall of an abscess, ulcer, etc.
       - b. Auto-immune or drug induced
       - c. Polyarteritis nodosa
       - d. Giant-cell arteritis
       - e. Thromboangiitis obliterans
2. Veins
   - (i) Inflammation (thrombophlebitis)
       - a. Trauma—fractures, tourniquets, i.v. catheters
       - b. Chemical—e.g. sclerosing fluids for treatment of varicose veins and haemorrhoids, irritant fluids administered intravenously
       - c. Bacterial infection, e.g. thrombophlebitis of venous sinuses complicating acute suppurative otitis media or mastoiditis

B. Changes in blood flow

1. Arteries
   Stasis and/or turbulence related to
   - (i) Aneurysms
   - (ii) Atherosclerotic plaques
   - (iii) Spasm

2. Veins
    (i)   Local causes
          a. Inactivity. Lack of muscular 'pumping' action greatly reduces venous flow
          b. Pressure on veins by ill-fitting plasters, bandages, gravid uterus, tumours, etc.
          c. Dilation and valvular incompetence, e.g. in varicose veins
    (ii) General factors
          a. Congestive cardiac failure
          b. Circulatory collapse following severe trauma, burns, etc.

C. Changes in the constitution of the blood
    1. Increased viscosity associated with erythraemia (or polycythaemia) promotes thrombosis in arteries and veins—due to:
        (i)   Dehydration, particularly in infancy leading to renal and cortical vein thrombosis
        (ii)   Chronic hypoxic states, e.g. respiratory failure, cyanotic congenital heart disease
        (iii) Polycythaemia rubra vera
    2. Hypercoaguable states found
        (i)   Following major surgery or trauma
        (ii)   In pregnancy and parturition
        (iii) In some users of the oral contraceptive pill
        (iv)   In some cases of leukaemia and polycythaemia rubra vera due to thrombocytosis
        (v)   After splenectomy
        (vi)   In endotoxaemia, shock, hypersensitivity reactions
        (vii) In association with some tumours e.g. carcinoma of the pancreas

STEPS IN THE FORMATION OF A THROMBUS

1. Deposition of platelets on the vascular endothelium as a result of
    (i)   Endothelial damage
    (ii)   Slowing of the blood flow
    (iii) Turbulence
2. Release of adenosine diphosphate (ADP) by the adherent platelets causes further platelet aggregation and deposition
3. Release of platelet thromboplastins and activation of Factor XII initiates coagulation. The consequent deposition of fibrin binds the platelet mass together
4. Fibrin formation continues with trapping of red blood cells
5. The rough surface of the developing thrombus acts as a stimulus for further platelet adhesion which is followed by deposition of another layer of fibrin and red blood cells

In this way, a laminated mass composed of alternating layers of platelet (pale) thrombus, and fibrin with enmeshed red blood cells (red thrombus) is built up. The irregular pale laminae are sometimes visible to the naked eye and are termed *lines of Zahn*. Once complete occlusion of the vessel has occurred, the static blood beyond the thrombus may undergo coagulation. Here coagulation is not occuring in circulating blood, and a homogeneous red *clot* is produced. In veins, the tail of this clot may reach a tributary vessel in which there is flowing blood and initiate a fresh thrombus. In this way, occlusion of small veins by thrombus and blood clot may extend proximally into major veins, a process termed *propagation*.

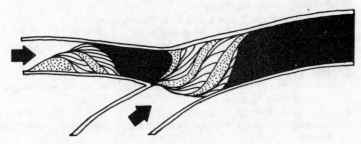

Propagation of thrombus in a vein

VENOUS THROMBOSIS
Venous thrombosis is much more common than thrombosis in arteries. It is increasing in frequency and is apparently related to the general prosperity of the population, being much less common in underdeveloped countries. The explanation for this might lie in differences in diet, in levels of activity, in longevity and in the number of surgical operations performed. Many thrombi are clinically 'silent'.

Factors implicated in venous thrombosis (phlebothrombosis)
1. Surgical operations. Thrombosis is common after operations
   (i) General effects, e.g. splenectomy
   (ii) Local effects, e.g. gynaecological and hip operations
   (iii) Loss of muscle 'pump' and direct pressure on veins during anaesthesia
   (iv) Immobilisation
2. Congestive cardiac failure and myocardial infarction. These are associated with venous stasis and immobilisation
3. Age. Thrombosis increases with age
4. Pregnancy
   (i) Hypercoaguable state
   (ii) Pressure on pelvic veins by gravid uterus
5. Oral contraceptive pill
6. Obesity
7. Malignancy, e.g. carcinoma of pancreas, possibly related to production of thromboplastins by the tumour cells

Location
1. Deep veins of the calf
2. Iliofemoral segment by propagation from the calf or arising *de novo*
3. Multiple sites simultaneously

Most venous thrombi are thought to originate in or close to a valve pocket.

Varieties of venous thrombosis
1. Thrombophlebitis—thrombosis secondary to inflammation of the vein wall
2. Thrombophlebitis migrans
   (i) Recurrent thrombosis at different sites
   (ii) Typically involves limb veins
   (iii) Often associated with visceral malignancy (Trousseau's sign)
3. Phlegmasia alba dolens—'painful white leg of pregnancy'—thrombosis of the femoral and external iliac veins associated with arterial spasm
4. Mondor's disease—Localised phlebitis affecting subcutaneous veins of the abdominal or thoracic wall, especially around the breast

ARTERIAL THROMBOSIS
Factors implicated in arterial thrombosis
1. Damage to the endothelial lining, e.g. atherosclerosis, trauma
2. Micro-turbulence around irregular atheromatous plaques
3. Major disturbances of flow in aneurysms or due to sustained spasm.

Types of thrombosis
1. Occluding thrombus in medium and small arteries frequently in association with concentric atherosclerosis
2. Thrombosis occurring over part of the wall of a large artery or the aorta—*mural* thrombosis

CARDIAC THROMBOSIS
Factors implicated in intracardiac thrombosis
1. Endocardial damage resulting from
   (i) Primary endocardial inflammation as in acute rheumatic fever
   (ii) Haemodynamic factors in chronic valvular disease and resultant mechanical injury
   (iii) Secondary to underlying myocardial damage as in myocardial infarction
2. Disordered contraction, e.g. intra-atrial thrombosis resulting from atrial fibrillation
3. Turbulence, as in a ventricular aneurysm following myocardial infarction

TYPES OF THROMBOSIS

1. Valvular thrombosis

Thrombi composed of platelets, fibrin and variable numbers of red blood cells formed on the valve cusps are termed *vegetations*. They are found in:

(i) Acute rheumatic fever. The vegetations (which are composed almost entirely of platelets) are small, compact, firm and rubbery.

(ii) Infective endocarditis. This condition affects valves previously damaged by rheumatic fever or congenitally abnormal valves e.g'. bicuspid aortic valve. The vegetations are large, friable, and contain the infective agent e.g. bacterial 'colonies' or more rarely, rickettsia, fungi and yeasts

(iii) Non-infective ('abacterial') thrombotic endocarditis. Known for many years as Lambl's excrescences, these sterile vegetations are found with increased frequency in patients with wasting diseases, particularly carcinomatosis. They are of variable size and may break off giving rise to cerebral ischaemia

(iv) Verrucous endocarditis (Libman-Sacks) found in some cases of systemic lupus erythematosus

2. Mural thrombosis

Thrombosis adherent to part of the endocardial lining is found in:

(i) Myocardial infarction which can result in inflammation of the endocardium and subsequent thrombosis

(ii) Rheumatic fever, MacCallum's patch in the left atrium resulting from mitral regurgitation

(iii) Acute myocarditis

3. Ball thrombus

A detached, ovoid or spherical thrombus may be formed in the atria in atrial fibrillation. This can impact in the mitral ring, for example, and produce a syncopal attack or even sudden death. More commonly, atrial fibrillation is associated with thrombosis in the atrial appendage or a polypoid thrombus attached to the wall.

FATE OF THROMBI

1. Resolution

The thrombus may be completely removed by a combination of:

(i) Shrinkage by a process analagous to clot-retraction *in vitro*

(ii) Fibrinolysis promoted by the release of plasminogen activator from the endothelium

(iii) Phagocytosis by macrophages which infiltrate the thrombus

2. Organisation

Ingrowth of endothelial cells, fibroblasts and smooth muscle cells convert the thrombus into fibrovascular tissue rich in collagen and elastin fibres.

(i) In occluding thrombi continuity of newly-formed vascular channels may be established and their subsequent dilatation lead to partial restoration of blood flow—a process known as *re-canalisation*

(ii) In mural thrombi the surface becomes re-endothelialised and the organised thrombus eventually becomes a fibrous plaque which may be indistinguishable from an atheromatous lesion

3. Detachment

A portion of a friable or loosely attached thrombus may break off into the circulation forming an *embolus*.

EMBOLISM

Embolism is the impaction in part of the vascular system of any abnormal undissolved material carried there by the blood stream. The recognised types are:

1. Thrombi
2. Fat embolism
3. Gaseous embolism
4. Tumour fragments
5. Infective agents
6. Atheromatous material
7. Amniotic fluid
8. Foreign bodies

1. Thrombi

These are by far the commonest type. The detached thrombus may be of venous, arterial, or cardiac origin.

Venous thrombosis in the leg or pelvic veins may lead to embolism to the pulmonary arteries. The possible results are:

(i) Sudden death after obstruction by major embolism resulting from
   a. Systemic anoxia
   b. Acute right ventricular failure
   c. ? Liberation of 5-HT causing spasm of the pulmonary arterial system
   d. ? Reflex vagal inhibition

(ii) Ischaemic necrosis of lung tissue, so-called *infarction*. In the lung, infarcts are haemorrhagic because of the dual blood supply (via pulmonary and bronchial arteries)

(iii) Progressive obliterative pulmonary hypertension from multiple microemboli

(iv) Arterial splits and aneurysms after acute stretching of the artery

Arterial and cardiac thrombosis

The main *sites* are:

- (i) Thrombus on atheromatous lesions in the aorta and major branches
- (ii) Vegetations on valves
- (iii) Mural thrombus in the left ventricle
- (iv) Atrial thrombus

Detachment results in:

- (i) Infarction of major organs, e.g. brain, kidney, spleen
- (ii) Arterial occlusion leading to gangrene of the intestine or limbs
- (iii) Large embolism lodging across the aortic bifurcation—'saddle' embolus, producing ischaemic changes in the lower limbs

2. Fat embolism

Is the impaction of large fat globules in small arteries and capillaries. It differs from thromboembolism in that the globules are fluid and deformable and so occlusion may be temporary or incomplete.

Causes of fat embolism

- (i) Fracture of long bones is the major cause
- (ii) Operative manipulation of fractures, e.g. in an arthroplasty
- (iii) Trauma to adipose tissue (rare)
- (iv) Trauma to a fatty liver (very rare)

Sites and effects

- (i) Pulmonary fat embolism
  - a. Minor degrees probably have little significance
  - b. More marked embolism is associated with hypoxaemia which may result from shunting of blood through pre-capillary anastomoses. Such shunting can also give rise to systemic embolism
- (ii) Systemic fat embolism is never found in the absence of pulmonary embolism. The most important site for impaction is the cerebral vasculature. This produces multiple small haemorrhagic and ischaemic lesions particulary in the white matter which may lead to coma and death. Multiple petechiae may be found in the skin

Origin of fat emboli

- (i) Trauma to fat cells releases globules of fat into the marrow veins, which then pass to the lungs
- (ii) ? Large fat globules form by fusion of chylomicrons under the influence of platelet factors released following trauma

3. Gaseous embolism

Causes
- (i) Mismanaged intravenous infusions
- (ii) Operations in which large veins are opened
- (iii) Air injections for radiological techniques
- (iv) Insufflation of the Fallopian tubes
- (v) Criminal abortion
- (vi) Caisson disease or decompression sickness (nitrogen bubbles forming as a consequence of rapid decompression)

Effects
- (i) Sudden death as a result of large volume of air reaching the right ventricle and preventing the propulsion of blood into the pulmonary artery
- (ii) Sudden decompression leads to tissue damage by bubble formation especially in the CNS ('diver's bends') and aseptic necrosis of bone resulting in osteoarthrosis

4. Tumour fragments
Vascular invasion is a common finding in malignant neoplasms, and clumps of tumour cells may detach and impact at some distant site. Whilst this may be a source of secondary tumours such embolism is rarely large enough to produce ischaemic damage. An exception is renal carcinoma where growth into the renal vein may give rise to relatively large tumour emboli.

5. Infective agents
- (i) Bacterial clusters, e.g. from infective endocarditis giving rise to pyaemic abscesses or 'mycotic' aneurysms
- (ii) Parasites, e.g. clumps of plasmodia in cerebral malaria

6. Atheromatous material
Rupture of the thin fibrous cap over a soft atheromatous plaque may lead to release of granular lipidic debris into the artery. This is a not uncommon cause of focal myocardial necrosis.

7. Amniotic fluid
Fluid may be driven through the placental bed into the maternal circulation during labour, particularly where there is obstruction.

Effects
- (i) Acute respiratory distress and shock which may be fatal
- (ii) Disseminated intravascular coagulation produced by thromboplastins in the fluid
- (iii) Afibrinogenaemia following plasmin activation

8. Foreign bodies

This is rare, but an important example is embolism of polythene catheters used in intravenous infusions which may break off and lodge in the heart.

Paradoxical embolism

The passage of an embolism from the right to the left side of the heart through a septal defect resulting in systemic arterial embolism from a venous source.

FURTHER READING

Morris, G.K. & Mitchell, J.R.A. (1977) The aetiology of acute pulmonary embolism and the identification of high risk groups. *British Journal of Hospital Medicine,* **18,** 6.

Nicolaides, A.N. (Ed.) (1975) *Thromboembolism : Aetiology, Advances in Prevention and Management.* Lancaster: Medical and Technical Publishing.

Sevitt, S. (1973) The mechanisms of canalisation in deep vein thrombosis. *Journal of Pathology,* **110,** 153.

Sevitt, S. (1973) The significance of fat embolism. *British Journal of Hospital Medicine,* **9,** 784.

Oedema and congestion

OEDEMA

Oedema is an excessive accumulation of fluid in the interstitial tissues or body cavities. Accumulations in the cavities are termed *ascites* (peritoneum), *hydrothorax* or *pleural effusion,* and *pericardial effusion.*

The fluid may be either an exudate or a transudate.

Exudate. High specific gravity ($>$1.020) fluid containing all the plasma proteins including fibrinogen and numerous inflammatory cells, and resulting from increased vascular permeability.

Transudate. Low specific gravity ($<$1.012) fluid containing small amounts of albumin and few cells. It arises from an imbalance in those forces tending to move fluid out of the vessels and those tending to retain it within them:

1. Forces moving fluid out of vessels
   (i)   Hydrostatic pressure of the blood
   (ii) Osmolarity of the interstitial fluid
2. Forces retaining fluid in the vessels
   (i)   Osmotic pressure of the plasma proteins
   (ii) Interstitial tissue pressure

Even when excessive quantities of fluid are passing out of vessels, increased lymphatic drainage may prevent the appearance of oedema. Conversely, lymphatic obstruction may itself produce oedema when the other factors are at normal levels.

Oedema may be generalised or localised.

A. Generalised oedema
1. Increased hydrostatic pressure of the blood
   (i)   Cardiac failure
2. Decreased osmotic pressure of the blood
   (i)   Excessive loss of protein
         a. Proteinuria, e.g. nephrotic syndrome
         b. Protein-losing enteropathy
   (ii) Inadequate synthesis of protein
         a. Hepatic cirrhosis
   (iii) Inadequate intake of protein
         a. Malnutrition (Kwashiorkor)
         b. Prolonged starvation
         c. Malabsorption syndromes

3. Increased osmostic pressure of the interstitial fluid due to sodium retention
   (i) Renal vasoconstriction and/or diminished glomerular filtration rate
      a. Cardiac failure
      b. Chronic renal disease
      c. Acute glomerulonephritis
   (ii) Increased levels of aldosterone secondary to:
      a. Cardiac failure
      b. Nephrotic syndrome
      c. Hepatic cirrhosis (failure of inactivation)
   (iii) Excess ACTH or cortisone
      a. Therapeutic
      b. Cushing's syndrome
4. Generalised increase in vascular permeability
   (i) Hypoxia
   (ii) Bacterial toxins
   (iii) Chemicals
5. Diminished tissue tension
   (i) Loss of elasticity with age
   (ii) Change in the ground substance, e.g. rendered more soluble by corticosteroids in Cushing's syndrome

B. Localised oedema
   1. Increased hydrostatic pressure of the blood due to:
      (i) Venous obstruction
         a. Venous thrombosis
         b. Strangulation/volvulus
         c. External pressure on veins—
            Gravid uterus
            Ligatures/Tourniquets
            Tumour
         d. Hepatic cirrhosis (portal hypertension)
      (ii) Gravity, e.g. ankle oedema after prolonged standing
   2. Increased vascular permeability
      (i) Chemical irritants giving rise to
         a. Urticarial reactions in skin
         b. Pulmonary oedema
      (ii) Immunological reactions with release of anaphylatoxins, including angioneurotic oedema
      (iii) Other causes of acute inflammation

ON

...d content of blood in an organ or tissue may be an
...eraemia in response to increased metabolic activity, for
...in skeletal muscle, or passive congestion.

...e congestion may result from local venous obstruction and
...s the formation of a transudate, or more frequently it is a
...quence of cardiac failure.

Cardiac failure can predominantly involve the right ventricle
giving rise to congestion of the abdominal organs together with
ascites and peripheral oedema, or involve the left ventricle
producing pulmonary congestion and under-perfusion of the
systemic circulation. Frequently, both ventricles are involved and a
state of congestive cardiac failure results.

Right ventricular failure (RVF)

Causes
1. Secondary to left ventricular failure
2. Pulmonary hypertension
3. Pulmonary embolism
4. Congenital heart disease
   (i) Atrial septal defect
   (ii) Pulmonary stenosis
   (iii) Tricuspid anomalies
5. Myocarditis
6. Myocardial infarction (rare in RV)

Effects of RVF
1. *Liver*
   (i) Hepatomegaly
   (ii) 'Nutmeg' appearance due to
       a. Centrilobular congestion and atrophy of liver cells
       b. Peripheral fatty change resulting from hypoxia
   (iii) Centrilobular necrosis in severe, acute congestion
   (iv) Centrilobular fibrosis in prolonged (chronic venous)
       congestion which may link up and give a false
       impression of cirrhosis. A true 'cardiac' cirrhosis, with
       regenerative nodules, is rare
2. *Spleen*
   (i) Mild to moderate splenomegaly
   (ii) Fibrosis of sinusoidal walls
   (iii) Haemosiderin deposition
3. *Kidneys*
   (i) Congestion
   (ii) Fatty change and/or cloudy swelling due to hypoxia
   (iii) Redistribution of blood flow with a relative increase to
       the medulla leading to sodium retention
4. *Oedema of the subcutaneous tissues*—mainly in the
   dependent parts of the body
5. *Brain*
   (i) Congestion
   (ii) Hypoxia
6. *Ascites due to portal congestion*

Left ventricular failure (LVF)

Causes
1. Systemic hypertension
2. Myocardial ischaemia (with or without infarction)
3. Rheumatic heart disease
   (i)   Mitral incompetence
   (ii) Aortic stenosis or incompetence
4. Calcific aortic stenosis
5. Coarctation of the aorta
6. Congenital heart disease
7. Cardiomyopathy
8. Myocarditis
9. High output states
   (i)   Pregnancy
   (ii)   Severe anaemia
   (iii) Hypoxia and hypercapnia
   (iv)   Pyrexia
   (v)   Thyrotoxicosis
   (vi)   Hepatic failure
   (vii) AV aneurysm
   (viii) Paget's disease
   (ix)   Beri-beri

Effects of LVF
1. Congestive effects in the lungs
   (i)   Pulmonary oedema
   (ii) Chronic venous congestion
         a. Capillary congestion
         b. Mild interstitial fibrosis mainly involving interlobular septa
         c. Intra-alveolar haemorrhage
         d. Haemosiderin-laden macrophages ('heart-failure cells')
   (iii) Pulmonary infarcts (especially in mitral stenosis)
   (iv) Hydrothorax
2. Effects of hypoperfusion
   (i)   Acute LVF may give rise to infarcts in organs where the blood supply is already compromised by atherosclerosis. They may be found in
         a. Kidneys
         b. Brain, particularly in 'watershed' areas
         c. Large intestine (ischaemic colitis/strictures)
   (ii) Kidney
         Decreased blood flow leads to:
         a. Hypoxia—hydropic vacuolation in tubular epithelium
         b. Diminished glomerular filtration rate resulting in salt and water retention

   (iii) Liver
       a. Centrilobular necrosis
       b. Fatty change
   (iv) Brain
        Individual cell necrosis in susceptible areas—the cornu ammonis and the Purkinje cell layer in the cerebellum

FURTHER READING

Slavin, G. *et al* (1975) Pulmonary oedema at necropsy: a combined pathological and radiological method of study. *Journal of Clinical Pathology,* **28**, 357.

Swan, H.J.C. & Parmley, W.W. (1974) Congestive heart failure. In *Pathologic Physiology,* 5th edn. ed. Sodeman, W.A. & Sodeman, W.A., p. 273. Philadelphia: Saunders.

The effects of injury on the body

GENERAL REACTIONS TO INJURY
1. Endocrine
   (i)   Increased secretion of ACTH, ADH, and growth hormone (in response to the early hypoglycaemia)
   (ii) Increased production of adrenal cortical hormones associated with 'compact-cell' change in the zona fasciculata
   (iii) Increased aldosterone production
   (iv) Increased production of catecholamines by the adrenal medulla in response to autonomic stimulation
   (v)   Increased production of thyroxine
2. Metabolic
   (i)   Initial hypoglycaemia
   (ii) Later hyperglycaemia resulting from increased glycogenolysis in the liver
   (iii) Negative nitrogen balance initially
   (iv) Hyperlipidaemia
   (v)   Moderate pyrexia
   (vi) Metabolic acidosis resulting from accumulation of lactate
3. Haematological
   (i)   Leucocytosis
   (ii) Lymphopenia
   (iii) Eosinopenia
   (iv) Thrombocytosis
4. Disseminated intravascular coagulation
   (i)   Hypercoagulability leading to microthrombosis
   (ii) Activation of fibrinolysis
   (iii) Consumption of platelets and coagulation factors
5. Electrolyte changes
   (i)   Increased potassium loss
   (ii) Sodium and water retention resulting from aldosterone secretion

COMPLICATIONS OF MAJOR TRAUMA
1. Haemorrhage and hypovolaemia
2. Traumatic shock (neurogenic/muscle injury)
3. Infection
4. Acute renal failure
5. Thromboembolism following venous thrombosis
6. Fat embolism
7. Disseminated intravascular coagulation

SHOCK
A state of circulatory failure leading to impaired perfusion of tissues with resultant hypoxic damage.

Pathogenesis
1. Hypovolaemia—a fall in cardiac output resulting from reduced blood volume
2. Cardiac failure—cardiogenic—a fall in output resulting from inadequate heart function ('pump failure')
3. Vascular mechanisms
    (i)   Pooling of blood in large peripheral vessels due to loss of vasomotor tone
    (ii)   Pooling of blood in capillaries resulting from persistent venular constriction
    (iii) Increased vascular permeability
    (iv)   Slowing of blood flow resulting from 'sludging' of red cells
    (v)   Disseminated intravascular coagulation

Causes
1. Hypovolaemia
    (i)   Haemorrhage
    (ii)   Loss of plasma, e.g. burns
    (iii) Loss of fluid and electrolytes, e.g. severe diarrhoea, diabetic keto-acidosis
2. Cardiogenic
    (i)   Myocardial infarction
    (ii)   Major pulmonary embolism
    (iii) Following cardiac surgery
    (iv)   Myocarditis and other causes of acute cardiac failure

3. Vascular
    (i)   Anaphylactic—Type I hypersensitivity
    (ii)   Neurogenic, e.g. spinal injuries
    (iii) Toxic—endotoxaemia

PATHOLOGICAL LESIONS IN SHOCK

1. Kidneys
   (i)   Acute tubular necrosis
   (ii) Glomerular microthrombosis
   (iii) Acute cortical necrosis (rare)
2. Lungs
   (i)   Congestion and oedema
   (ii) Microthrombi
   (iii) Hyaline-membrane formation
   (iv) Atelectasis
3. Liver
   (i)   Centrilobular necrosis
   (ii) Fatty change
4. Adrenals
   (i)   Compact-cell change in cortex
   (ii) Focal necrosis of cortical cells
   (iii) Massive haemorrhage (Waterhouse-Friderichsen syndrome)
5. Heart
   (i)   Fatty change
   (ii) Subendocardial haemorrhage
6. Gastrointestinal tract
   (i)   Acute ulceration of the stomach and duodenum usually associated with severe burns (Curling's ulcers)
   (ii) Haemorrhagic gastroenteropathy
         Focal or more extensive haemorrhage into the intestinal mucosa associated with local superficial ulceration, probably resulting from hypoxia
7. Brain
   Anoxic or hypoxic encephalopathy
8. Pituitary
   Necrosis following hypovolaemia (most commonly due to post-partum haemorrhage) giving rise to:
   (i)   Acute insufficiency—Sheehan's syndrome
   (ii) Chronic insufficiency—Simmond's disease

FURTHER READING

Hunt, A.C. (Ed.) (1972) *Pathology of Injury.* Report and Recommendations of a Working Party of the Royal College of Pathologists. Aylesbury: Harvey, Miller & Medcalf.

Sevitt, S. (1972) Physiology and pathology of injury. *The Pathological Basis of Medicine,* ed. Curran, R.C. & Harnden, D.G. p. 281. London: Heinemann.

Congenital malformations

Congenital malformations are primary defects in body structure resulting from an error of morphogenesis. They are to be distinguished from *deformations* which are alterations in shape and/or structure of a previously normally formed part, e.g. congenital torticollis, congenital postural scoliosis, talipes (deformities of the feet), etc. Major congenital defects are found in about 2.5% of total births, and of these, neural-tube defects, such as spina bifida and anencephaly, and congenital heart disease each account for about one third.

CAUSES OF CONGENITAL MALFORMATION
1. **Environmental factors**
   (i)   Nutritional disturbances
         Experimental studies have demonstrated the importance of essential vitamins (vitamin A, riboflavin, folic acid) but clinical proof is lacking
   (ii) Maternal infection
         a. Rubella
         b. Cytomegalovirus
         c. Toxoplasmosis
         Malformations have also been described after influenza, measles, mumps, polio, *echo* and coxsackie infections. These are all rare associations and a causal relationship has not been proven
   (iii) Hormonal agents
         a. Masculinisation of females has resulted from administration of androgens or progesterone in early pregnancy, or as a result of congenital adrenal hyperplasia
         b. Insulin used in treatment of maternal diabetes may lead to malformation (?)
         c. Hypoplasia of the adrenals results from pituitary deficiency in anencephaly
   (iv) Drugs
         a. Thalidomide (limb defects)
         b. Anti-metabolites
         c. Other commonly used drugs, e.g. salicylates, sulphonamides, and streptomycin, have had *teratogenic* effects in animals, but evidence in humans is lacking

    (v)   Mechanical factors
             Compression of the fetus is important in producing
             deformations, and may exaggerate the deformities
             associated with malformations, e.g. in congenital
             dislocation of the hip
    (vi)   Irradiation
    (vii) Hypoxia—may lead to cardiac malformations in children
             born at high altitudes
   (viii) Disordered circulation in the embryo
    (ix)   Maternal age and birth rank
           a. Mongolism
           b. Hydrocephalus
           c. Achondroplasia
           d. Anencephaly
           are more frequent with increasing maternal age

2. Single gene defects

Malformations with autosomal dominant inheritance include:
    (i)   Achondroplasia
    (ii)   Brachydactyly/polydactyly/syndactyly
    (iii) Mandibulo-facial dysostosis (Treacher-Collins)
    (iv) Cranio-cleidal dysostosis
    (v)   Congenital dislocation of the hip
    (vi) Ehlers-Danlos syndrome (hyperelastosis cutis)

3. Chromosome abnormalities

Autosomal anomalies
    (i)   Trisomy 21, Down's syndrome (mongolism)
           a. Characteristic facies
           b. Macroglossia
           c. Single transverse palmar crease
           d. Cardiac lesions:
               Atrial septal defect
               Ventricular septal defect
               Patent ductus
               Tetralogy of Fallot
           e. Duodenal atresia
    (ii)   Trisomy 17–18
           a. Skull deformed
           b. Low-set ears
           c. Micrognathos
           d. Flexion deformities of the fingers
           e. 'Rocker-bottom' foot deformity
    (iii) Cri-du-chat syndrome (short arm of chromosome 5)
           a. Microcephaly
           b. Widely separated eyes
           c. Characteristic cry
           d. Hypotonia
           e. CVS malformations

Sex chromosome anomalies

   (i)   45 XO (Turner's syndrome)
      a. Dwarfism
      b. Sexual infantilism
      c. Increased carrying angle of lower arms
      d. Webbed neck
      e. Broad chest with widely-spaced nipples
      f. Streaked gonads in position of ovaries
  (ii)   47 XXX   Some loss of intelligence
 (iii)   47 XXY (Klinefelter)   and infertility
 (iv)   48 XXXY
  (v)   48 XXXXY
      a. Mental retardation
      b. Minute testes
      c. Dwarfism
      d. Congenital heart disease
      e. Radioulnar synostosis
 (vi)   47 XYY—tall, aggressive males who may show
      a. Sexual maldevelopment
      b. Skeletal disorders
      c. Myopia
      d. Marfan's syndrome

FURTHER READING

Insley, J. (1970) Sex chromosome abnormalities in children. *British Journal of Medicine,* **4**, 103.

Pitcher, D.R. (1971) The XYY syndrome. *British Journal of Hospital Medicine,* **5**, 279.

Warkany, J. (1971) *Congenital Malformations.* New York: Year Book Medical Publishers.

Inborn errors of metabolism

When a genetic error results in the formation of an abnormal protein, and this protein is an enzyme, the resultant biochemical defect may become manifest through the accumulation of some precursor or substrate which brings about a disease syndrome. Such diseases, usually inherited as Mendelian recessives, are termed inborn errors of metabolism. They can be grouped into four main categories involving:

A. Errors of carbohydrate metabolism
B. Errors of amino-acid metabolism
C. Errors of lysosomal function
D. Errors of steroid metabolism

A. Errors of carbohydrate metabolisim
include:

1. Galactosaemia (deficiency of galactose-1-phosphate uridyl transferase)— results in:
   (i) Vomiting and diarrhoea
   (ii) Ascites
   (iii) Hepato-splenomegaly
   (iv) Jaundice
   (v) Fatty change in the liver with pseudo-glandular rosettes of hepatocytes
   (vi) Cataracts

2. Glycogen storage diseases include:

Type	Enzyme deficient
I (von Gierke's)	Glucose-6-phosphatase
II (Pompe's)	α-1, 4, 6 glucosidase (see p. 103)
III (Limit dextrinosis)	Amylo-1, 6-glucosidase (debrancher)
IV	Amylo-1, 4-1, 6-transglucosidase (brancher)
V (McArdle's)	Muscle phosphorylase
VI	Liver phosphorylase
VII	Glycogen synthetase

3. Fructose intolerance (fructose -1-phosphate aldolase)

B. Errors of amino acid metabolism
include:
1. Phenylketonuria (phenylalanine hydroxylase deficiency resulting in accumulation of phenylalanine)
   Results
   (i)   Reduced hair and skin pigmentation
   (ii) Dermatitis (variable)
   (iii) Myoclonus
   (iv) Mental deficiency
2. Tyrosinosis (*p*-hydroxyphenylpyruvic acid oxidase deficiency resulting in accumulation of phenylalanine and tyrosine) May be transient, or permanent as part of a syndrome associated with
   (i)   Renal tubular defects
   (ii) Vitamin D-resistant rickets
   (iii) Cirrhosis
3. Alkaptonuria (homogentisic acid oxidase)
   Ochronosis-deposition of homogentisic acid in cartilage and other tissues
   Results
   (i)   Pigmentation of face, ears and sclerae
   (ii) Arthritis
4. Maple syrup urine disease (branched-chain ketoacid decarboxylase deficiency resulting in accumulation of α-ketoacids)
   Results
   (i)   Dysphagia
   (ii) Areflexia
   (iii) Mental deficiency
5. Homocystinuria (cystathione synthetase deficiency)
   (i)   Dislocation of the lens
   (ii)   Cataracts
   (iii) Genu valgum
   (iv)   Arachnodactyly
   (v)   Spastic paraplegia
   (vi)   Brittle hair
   (vii) Thromboembolic disease
   (viii) Osteoporosis
   (ix)   Mental retardation

C. Errors in lysosomal function
leading to

1. *Accumulation of sphingolipids*

   (*see* table opposite.)

Disease	Lipid stored	Enzyme defect
(i) Tay Sach's	GM_2 gangliosides	Hexosaminidase A

   a. Progressive optic atrophy
   b. Cherry-red spot at the macula
   c. Generalised spasticity

(ii) Generalised gangliosidosis	GM_1 ganglioside	ß-galactosidase

   a. Psycho-motor deterioration
   b. Hepatomegaly
   c. Bony deformities

(iii) Krabbe's Mental retardation	Galactosyl ceramide	ß-Galactosidase

(iv) Gaucher's	Glucosyl ceramide	ß-Glucosidase

   a. Acute type in infancy with
      gross hepato/splenomegaly
   b. Chronic type in adults with
      skin pigmentation
      hepato/splenomegaly and
      hypersplenism, and bone pain

(v) Niemann-Pick's	Sphingomyelin	Sphingomyelinase

   a. Hepato/splenomegaly
   b. CNS involvement resulting in
      mental deterioration

(vi) Metachromatic leucodystrophy

	Cerebroside sulphate	Specific sulphatidase

   a. Dementia
   b. Neuropathy with extrinsic
      ocular muscle paralysis
   c. Optic atrophy

(vii) Anderson-Fabry's	Trihexosyl ceramide	Ceramide trihexosidase

   a. Fever and arthralgia
   b. Angiokeratoma corporis
      diffusum universale (diffuse
      ectasia and tortuosity of small
      blood vessels)
   c. Proteinuria and renal failure

(viii)Fucosidosis	Fucoglycolipid	α-L-fucosidase

2. *Accumulation of neutral lipids*

Disease	Lipid stored	Enzyme defe
(i) Wolman's	Triglyceride cholesterol esters	Acid esterase

a. Diarrhoea
  b. Hepatomegaly
  c. Calcification of the adrenals		

(ii) Cholesterol ester storage a. Hepatomegaly	Cholesterol ester	?

(iii) Cerebro-tendinous xanthomatosis
  a. Tendon xanthomata
  b. Cataracts
  c. Cerebellar ataxia
	Cholesterol esters	?

3. *Accumulation of glycosaminoglycans (mucopolysaccharidoses)*

Disease	Compound stored or excreted in excess	Enzyme defect
I H (Hurler)	Dermatan sulphate Heparan sulphate	α-L-iduronidase
I S (Scheie)	Dermatan sulphate	α-L-iduronidase
II (Hunter)	Dermatan sulphate Heparan sulphate	L-iduronosulphate sulphatase
IIIA (Sanfilippo) IIIB (Sanfillipo)	Heparan sulphate with or without dermatan sulphate	Heparan sulphate sulphamidase α-N-acetylglucoraminidase
IV (Morquio)	Keratan sulphate Chondroitin-6-sulphate	N-acetyl hexosamine-4-sulphate sulphatase
VI (Maroteaux-Lamy)	Dermatan sulphate	Arylsulphatase-B

Most of these diseases are characterised by stunting of growth and mental deterioration, with variable facial deformity, hepato-splenomegaly, and heart and bone involvement.

4. Accumulation of other compounds

Disease	Compound stored	Enzyme defect
(i) Refsum's	Phytanic acid	Phytanic acid oxidase

   a. Nerve deafness
   b. Peripheral neuropathy
   c. Icthyosis ('fish-scale' skin)
   d. Cerebellar ataxia
   e. Retinitis pigmentosa

(ii) Cystinosis (Lignac-Fanconi)	Cystine	?

   a. Hepato-splenomegaly
   b. Renal tubular acidosis
   c. Progressive renal failure
   d. Renal rickets

(iii) Pompe's disease	Glycogen	Lysosomal-α-glucosidase

   a. Muscle weakness at, or soon after, birth
   b. Cardiomegaly
   c. Macroglossia
   d. Mild hepatomegaly with intra-lysosomal glycogen accumulation

5. Other lysosomal enzyme disorders
   (i)   Hyperphosphatasia resulting from an excess of alkaline phosphatase
         a. Mental retardation
         b. Cataracts
   (ii) Hypophosphatasia
         a. Failure to thrive
         b. Premature synostosis of the skull
         c. Metastatic calcification including nephrocalcinosis
         d. Faulty calcification of bone
   (iii) Acid phosphatase deficiency
         a. Vomiting
         b. Progressive CNS deterioration

D. Errors of steroid metabolism
Resulting in congenital adrenal hyperplasia

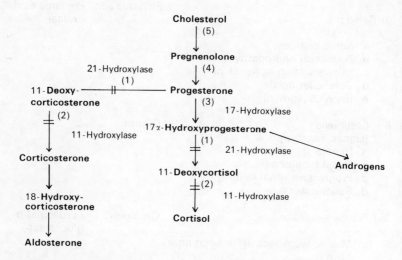

The principal defects are:
1. 21-Hydroxylase deficiency resulting in
    (i) Virilism
    (ii) Salt losing crises
2. 11-Hydroxylase deficiency
    (i) Hypertension resulting from excessive production of deoxycorticosterone and other mineralocorticoids
    (ii) Salt and water retention
    (iii) Virilisation
Other enzymes may be involved, these are:
3. 17-Hydroxylase
4. 3 ß-Hydroxysteroid dehydrogenase
5. Desmolase

FURTHER READING

Emery, A.E.H. (1971) *Elements of Medical Genetics,* 2nd edn. Edinburgh: E. & S. Livingstone.

Hers, H.G. & van Hoof, F. (Eds.) (1973) *Lysosomes and Storage Diseases.* London: Academic Press.

Raine, D.N. (Ed.) (1974) Molecular variants in disease. *Journal of Clinical Pathology,* **27,** Suppl. 5.

Stanbury, J.B., Wyngaarden, J.B. & Fredrickson, D.S. (1972) *The Metabolic Basis of Inherited Disease,* 3rd edn. New York: McGraw-Hill.

Disorders of body pigments

HAEMOGLOBIN

Haemoglobin is a conjugated protein composed of four haem groups attached to globin. Haem consists of a tetrapyrrole (porphyrin) ring with a ferrous ion at its centre.

Haemoglobin from effete red cells is normally broken down in reticuloendothelial cells of the spleen, bone marrow, and liver. The protein moiety is detached and broken down into its constituent amino acids which are re-metabolised. The iron combines with a ß-globulin apoferritin to form ferritin which in turn is bound to the globulin transferrin and transported in the plasma. The porphyrin moiety is converted into bilirubin and excreted.

Apart from the inherited disorders of globin synthesis (the haemoglobinopathies), haemoglobin and its products are subject to the following disturbances:

A. Disordered synthesis of haem resulting from abnormal porphyrin metabolism
B. Formation of abnormal haemoglobin compounds
C. Abnormal bilirubin metabolism and excretion leading to hyperbilirubinaemia
D. Abnormal storage of iron

A. **Porphyrin metabolism and its abnormalities**
Normal haem synthesis

Glycine + Succinyl – Coenzyme A

$\downarrow$ δ-aminolaevulate synthetase **(ALA-S)**

δ-Aminolaevulinic acid (ALA)

$\downarrow$

Porphobilinogen (PBG)

$\downarrow$

Uroporphyrinogen → Uroporphrin

$\downarrow$

Coproporphyrinogen → Coproporphyrin ⎤ **Excreted**

$\downarrow$

Protoporphyrinogen → Protoporphyrin + Fe^{++}

$\downarrow$

Haem

1. *Disordered synthesis in the liver* (hepatic porphyrias)
    (i)   Inherited as autosomal dominants
        a. Acute intermittent porphyria
        b. Porphyria variegata (South African type)
        c. Hereditary coproporphyria
  Mechanism
  ?   Increased activity of ALA-S in response to a partial
      blockage of haem formation operating at different points
      in its synthesis for each disease
  Results
        a. Acute abdominal pain
        b. Neuro-psychiatric attacks
        c. Excretion of large quantities of PBG and ALA in the
          urine. The attacks may be precipitated by drugs,
          especially barbiturates
    (ii)   Sporadic—symptomatic cutaneous hepatic porphyria.
        This is usually a consequence of chronic liver disease,
        especially chronic alcoholism
  Results
        a. Skin photosensitivity
        b. Hypermelanosis
        c. Hypertrichosis
        d. Excretion of large quantities of red-coloured
          uroporphyrin in the urine

2. *Disordered synthesis in the bone marrow* (erythropoietic
porphyrias)
    (i)   Congenital erythropoietic porphyria (recessive)
  Results
        a. Bulla formation in the skin in response to light and
          trauma
        b. Accumulations of uro- and coproporphyrins in the
          bone marrow, red blood cells and teeth
        c. Excess excretion of uro- and coproporphyrins in the
          urine and faeces
    (ii)   Erythropoietic protoporphyria (dominant)
        a. Photosensitivity of the skin but no bullae in response
          to trauma
        b. Increased amounts of protoporphyrin in red cells and
          faeces but not in the urine
    (iii) Erythropoietic coproporphyria
        a. Photosensitivity
        b. Increased coproporphyrins in faeces

B. Abnormal haemoglobin compounds

1. Carboxyhaemoglobin resulting from combination with carbon monoxide and producing a characteristic cherry-red colour in the blood
2. Methaemoglobin results from the conversion of the ferrous to a ferric ion, and in this form cannot combine with oxygen
    (i) Congenital—due to either a haemoglobinopathy (Hb-M) or a deficiency of methaemoglobin reductase (diaphorase)
    (ii) Acquired—drug-induced—due to phenacetin, sulphonamides, nitrates, and other oxidising drugs
3. Sulphaemoglobin—drug-induced—due to phenacetin, acetanilide

C. Hyperbilirubinaemia (jaundice)

Normal bilirubin metabolism and excretion

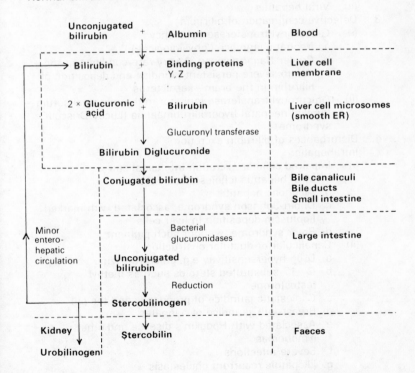

Unconjugated bilirubin + Albumin		Blood
Bilirubin + Binding proteins Y, Z		Liver cell membrane
2 × Glucuronic acid + Bilirubin		Liver cell microsomes (smooth ER)
Glucuronyl transferase		
Bilirubin Diglucuronide		
Conjugated bilirubin		Bile canaliculi Bile ducts Small intestine
Minor entero-hepatic circulation	Bacterial glucuronidases	Large intestine
Unconjugated bilirubin		
Reduction		
Stercobilinogen		
Kidney — Stercobilin		Faeces
Urobilinogen		

Causes of jaundice
1. Excessive bilirubin production overloading the conjugating
    capacity of the liver
    (i)   Haemolysis due to
           a. Hereditary spherocytosis
           b. Hereditary red-cell enzyme defects
           c. Thalassaemia
           d. Sickle-cell disease
           e. Auto-immune haemolytic anaemia
           f. Secondary to Hodgkin's disease, leukaemias, etc.
    (ii)   Increased production by the bone marrow—primary
           'shunt' hyperbilirubinaemia
2. Decreased uptake of bilirubin into liver cells and transport to
    the smooth endoplasmic reticulum
    (i)   Gilbert's disease. A familial condition resulting in mild
           intermittent jaundice
    (ii)   Viral hepatitis
3. Defective conjugation of bilirubin
    (i)   Glucuronyl transferase deficiency
           a. Neonatal jaundice ('physiological')
           b. Crigler-Najjar disease. A very rare condition giving
               rise to severe persistent jaundice and deposition of
               bilirubin in the brain—kernicterus
    (ii)   Glucuronyl transferase inhibitor in the maternal serum—
           familial neonatal hyperbilirubinaemia (Lucey-Driscoll
           syndrome)

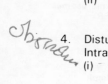

4. Disturbances of bilirubin excretion
    Intrahepatic:
    (i)   Impaired cellular excretion into canaliculi
           a. Viral hepatitis (cholestatic type)
           b. Alcoholic hepatitis
           c. Dubin-Johnson syndrome, associated with marked
               lipofuscin deposition in liver cells
           d. Rotor syndrome, without such pigment
    (ii)   Canalicular or ductular obstruction
           a. Drug hypersensitivity e.g. chlorpromazine
           b. C - 17 substituted steroids such as methyl
               testosterone
           c. Cholestatic jaundice of pregnancy and the pill
           d. Breast-milk jaundice of neonates
           e. Associated with Hodgkin's disease and other
               lymphomas
           f. Severe infections
           g. Idiopathic recurrent cholestasis
    (iii) Bile duct obstruction
           a. Primary biliary cirrhosis
           b. Sclerosing cholangitis
           c. Intrahepatic biliary atresia
           d. Cholangiocarcinoma

Extrahepatic bile duct obstruction
(i)   Gall-stones
(ii)   Carcinoma of the pancreas/ampulla
(iii) Pressure by tumour involved lymph glands at the porta
        hepatis
(iv)   Sclerosis of the extrahepatic ducts
(v)   Postoperative stricture

5. Hepatic failure
The jaundice of hepatic failure may result from several
disturbances but the principal defect is that there are
insufficient functioning liver cells to conjugate the normal
bilirubin load. The major *causes* are:
(i)   Terminal cirrhosis
(ii)   Massive necrosis
        a. Fulminant viral hepatitis
        b. Drug hepatotoxicity, e.g. paracetamol overdosage,
           halothane hepatitis

D. Abnormal storage of iron

Iron is normally stored as ferritin or as haemosiderin, which
consists of partly denatured ferritin. When excessive quantities
require to be stored clumps of haemosiderin appear in the tissues
and can be readily demonstrated by the Prussian Blue reaction.
Haemosiderin deposition may be localised or generalised:

1. Localised deposits are found in:
    (i)   Areas of haemorrhage in haemosiderin-laden
            macrophages
    (ii)   Renal tubular cells in haemoglobinuria
    (iii) Siderotic nodules (Gamna-Gandy bodies) in
            splenomegaly with hepatic cirrhosis.

2. Generalised deposition may result from:
    (i)   Excessive absorption of iron from the diet due to
            a. An inborn error of metabolism
            b. A greatly increased dietary intake
            c. In thalassaemia, sideroblastic anaemia, and
               spherocytosis (in the absence of transfusions)

Prolonged increased absorption leads to complete saturation of
circulating transferrin and thereafter absorbed iron is present in
portal blood in the unbound form. Free iron is toxic and produces
chronic cell injury in the liver resulting in cirrhosis. With the
development of vascular shunts in the cirrhotic liver, free iron
enters the systemic circulation and affects other organs, notably the
heart and pancreas. A variety of functional disturbances may ensue
and this parenchymatous iron storage disease is *haemochromatosis*.

    (ii)   Excessive administration of iron by multiple transfusions
            or parenteral injections

This usually results in iron deposition in macrophages of the bone
marrow, liver, and spleen and is termed *haemosiderosis*. If
administration is prolonged or massive amounts are given, then
saturation followed by parenchymatous deposition and fibrosis may
result in a picture indistinguishable from haemochromatosis.

Haemochromatosis may affect many organs

a. Liver—producing cirrhosis which in turn is associated with an increased incidence of hepatocellular carcinoma
b. Pancreas—interacinar fibrosis with pigmentation and atrophy of islets leading to diabetes mellitus
c. Skin—increase in melanin in the basal layer of the epidermis. Haemosiderin is also present mainly around skin appendages
d. Heart—pigmentation and atrophy of myocardial fibres resulting in arrhythmias and cardiac failure
e. Stomach—rare cases show deposition of haemosiderin in chief cells of the gastric mucosa but the pigment has little effect on pepsin secretion
f. Spleen—pigmentation and fibrosis
g. There may be pigmentation and atrophy in testes, thyroid, adrenals and pituitary

MELANIN

In the skin melanin is produced by single-cell 'glands', the *melanocytes,* which pass the pigment granules (*melanosomes*) to adjacent epidermal cells via their fine dendritic processes. Melanocytes appear as pale vacuolated cells scattered along the basal layer in H & E sections. The dendritic processes can be demonstrated using silver stains. These cells were formerly thought to originate from modified basal cells, but it is now generally accepted that they originate from precursor cells (*melanoblasts*) derived from the neural crest. During early fetal life these cells migrate into the dermis along with the nerves of the skin and then pass into the epidermis where they mature.

The melanocyte contains several enzymes, the most important in regard to pigment production being *tyrosinase* which converts tyrosine to melanin. In some circumstances the demonstration of tyrosinase activity can be an aid to diagnosis, for example, where a suspected malignant melanoma does not contain melanin. Frozen sections of the lesion are incubated with substrate (usually dihydroxyphenylalanine—DOPA, which gives faster results than tyrosine) and tyrosinase activity is indicated by the development of melanin pigment in the cell cytoplasm.

A. Lack of pigmentation
1. Genetic/naevoid causes
   (i)   Vitiligo
   (ii)   Piebaldism
   (iii) Albinism
   (iv)   Phenylketonuria
   (v)   Tuberous sclerosis
   (vi)   Naevus depigmentosus

2. Acquired causes
   (i) Endocrine
      a. Panhypopituitarism (lack of MSH)
      b. Hypoparathyroidism—moniliasis syndrome
      c. Male eunuchoidism
   (ii) Pernicious anaemia
   (iii) Postinflammatory
      a. Eczema
      b. Psoriasis
      c. Leprosy
   (iv) Chemicals/drugs
      a. Hydroquinone
      b. Chloroquine
      c. Phenolic disinfectants
   (v) Neoplasms
      a. Halo naevus
      b. Depigmentation of skin surrounding some malignant
         melanomas

B. Excessive pigmentation
1. Genetic/naevoid causes
   (i) Freckles
   (ii) Neurofibromatosis (*café au lait* spots)
   (iii) Generalised or focal lentigines
   (iv) Peutz-Jeghers syndrome—macular pigmentation of lips
        and buccal mucosa associated with polyposis of the
        small intestine
   (v) Albright's syndrome—pigmentation, fibrous dysplasia in
       bones, and sexual precocity
   (vi) Xeroderma pigmentosum
2. Acquired causes
   (i) Physical agents,
      a. Ultraviolet light (sun-tan)
      b. Ionising radiation
      c. Heat
   (ii) Endocrine
      a. Addison's disease
      b. ACTH-, and MSH-producing tumours
      c. ACTH therapy
      d. Pregnancy and contraceptive pill (facial
         pigmentation—'chloasma' due to excessive
         oestrogens)
      e. Thyrotoxicosis
   (iii) Metabolic
      a. Porphyrias
      b. Chronic liver disease
      c. Haemochromatosis
   (iv) Nutritional
      a. Chronic malnutrition—cachexia
      b. Pellagra

(v)   Rheumatoid arthritis, particularly Felty's syndrome
(vi)   Amyloidosis
(vii) Scleroderma
(vii) Chemicals/drugs
    a. Arsenic
    b. Chlórpromazine
(ix)   Neoplasms
    a. Malignant melanoma
    b. Acanthosis nigricans with underlying carcinoma
      (usually adenocarcinoma of the stomach)

C. Pigmentation by dermal melanocytes
1. Mongolian blue spot—bluish pigmentation found in the lumbosacral region which fades with increasing age
2. Blue naevus—elongated dendritic cells contain abundant melanin in the middle and deep dermis
3. Oculodermal melanosis (Naevus of Ota)—periorbital pigmentation by more superficially situated melanocytes

LIPOFUSCINS

These are widely distributed brown-pigments derived from the oxidation of lipids and are of heterogeneous composition. The pigment is seen in the following situations:
1. In certain apparently normal cells
    (i)   Epithelial cells of the epididymis
    (ii)   Interstitial cells of the testis
    (iii) Ganglion cells and neurones
2. In ageing cells—so-called 'wear-and-tear' pigment. This is best seen in 'permanent' tissues such as myocardium where the fibres show increasing pigmentation with age. It is particularly evident where the heart has atrophied as a result of wasting diseases—'brown atrophy'
3. As 'ceroid' pigment in the liver after liver cell necrosis and oxidation of lipidic membranes, e.g. after viral hepatitis, drug hepatotoxicity
4. In liver cells in the Dubin-Johnson syndrome
5. In the 'brown-bowel' syndrome. Pigmentation of smooth muscle cells accompanies various malabsorption states.

FURTHER READING

Bleehen, S.S. (1975) Disorders of melanin pigmentation. *British Journal of Hospital Medicine,* **13,** 590.
Wolman, M. (Ed.) (1969) *Pigments in Pathology.* London: Academic Press.

Calcification

Calcification other than that normally occuring in the teeth and skeletal system (*heterotopic calcification*) is seen in the following circumstances:

1. Associated with advancing age
    Deposits are found in:
    (i)   Pineal gland
    (ii) Tracheal and laryngeal cartilages
    (iii) Costal cartilages
2. In dead or degenerate tissue (*dystrophic calcification*)
    Examples
    (i)   In old tuberculous lesions
    (ii) In scars
    (iii) In dead parasites
    (iv) In degenerate tumours, especially uterine leiomyomata (fibroids)
    (v)   In atheromatous plaques
3. In association with increased levels of calcium (or occasionally with increased phosphate) in the blood and tissues, usually derived from the skeleton but also including increased absorption from the intestine. Such calcification occurs in previously normal tissues and is referred to as *metastatic*. It is found in:
    (i)   Hyperparathyroidism
          Primary, due to:
          a. Adenoma
          b. Hyperplasia
          c. Carcinoma (very rarely)
          Secondary, due to:
          a. Chronic renal failure
          b. Renal tubular acidosis
          c. Malabsorption states
          d. Pregnancy and lactation
    (ii) Malignancy with or without skeletal involvement
    (iii) Myelomatosis
    (iv) Vitamin D sensitivity, as in sarcoidosis and infantile hypercalcaemia
    (v)   Excessive administration of vitamin D
    (vi) Paget's disease of bone, (when immobilised)
    (vii) Hypophosphatasia
    (vii) Milk-alkali syndrome
    (ix) Hypoparathyroidism (deposits in the basal ganglia)

Sites of metastatic calcification
(i)   Kidneys, producing nephrocalcinosis which may lead to renal failure
(ii)   Stomach
(iii)   Lungs, on the elastic fibres of the alveolar septa
(iv)   Blood vessels
(v)   Cornea
4. In calculi (stones)
Many calculi include calcium salts among their constituents. Calculi are found in:
(i)   Urinary tract
a. calcium phosphate
b. calcium oxalate
c. calcium carbonate
(ii)   Biliary system
a. calcium bilirubinate
(iii)   Salivary glands
(iv)   Pancreas
(v)   Prostate
5. In neoplasia
Microscopic laminated calcified bodies—*calcospherites* are found in association with:
a. Adenocarcinoma of the ovary
b. Papillary carcinoma of the thyroid
c. Meningioma (psammoma bodies)
d. Benign and malignant breast lesions
e. Oligodendroglioma

FURTHER READING

Bickel, H. & Stern, J. (Eds.) (1976) *Inborn Errors of Calcium and Bone Metabolism.* Lancaster: Medical and Technical Publishing.
Schraer, H. (Ed.) (1970) *Biological Calcification: Cellular and Molecular Aspects.* London: North-Holland.

Amyloid

Amyloid appears as a homogeneous eosinophilic hyaline material under the light microscope and is found as an extracellular deposit in a wide variety of conditions.

FORMS OF AMYLOID DEPOSITION

A. *Systemic amyloidosis* associated with some predisposing disease (*secondary*).
1. Chronic infection (of long standing)
   (i) Tuberculosis
   (ii) Bronchiectasis
   (iii) Osteomyelitis
   (iv) Leprosy
   (v) Syphilis
2. Chronic inflammatory diseases
   (i) Rheumatoid arthritis
   (ii) Ulcerative colitis
   (iii) Systemic lupus erythematosus
   (iv) Pustular psoriasis
3. Abnormal proliferation of plasma cells
   (i) Multiple myeloma
   (ii) Waldenstrom's macroglobulinaemia
4. Associated with other neoplasms
   (i) Hodgkin's disease
   (ii) Carcinomas of bladder, kidney, stomach, bronchus, ovary

B. *Systemic amyloidosis* not associated with a known predisposing condition (*primary*)

C. *Hereditary/familial types*
   (i) Amyloidosis associated with Mediterranean fever
   (ii) Amyloid cardiomyopathy
   (iii) Amyloid polyneuropathy
   (iv) Familial amyloid nephropathy, urticaria and deafness
   (v) Familial cutaneous amyloid

D. *Localised* amyloid deposition
  (i) As an ageing phenomenon in the heart, brain (in senile
       plaques, and in the walls of small cerebral blood vessels)
       islets of Langerhans, and seminal vesicles
  (ii) In the stroma of certain tumours
       a. Medullary carcinoma of the thyroid
       b. Pituitary adenoma
       c. Islet-cell tumours of the pancreas
       These tumours are of APUD-cell origin, cells derived
       from the neuroectoderm which are distributed
       throughout the GI and respiratory tract and certain
       endocrine organs, and are capable of Amine-Precursor-
       Uptake and Decarboxylation. The stromal deposits are
       sometimes referred to as APUD-amyloid
       d. Basal cell carcinoma
  (iii) In the islets of Langerhans in diabetes mellitus
  (iv) As tumour-like deposits in:
       a. Larynx, trachea, bronchi and lung
       b. Genitourinary tract
       c. Eye
       d. Tongue
       e. Heart
       f. Skin

NATURE OF AMYLOID

Amyloid consists of protein arranged in fibrils. The protein (ml.wt
5000 – 18300) is composed of amino acids in an arrangement
which in some cases is identical to the sequence found in amino-
terminal light-chains of immunoglobulin, mainly of lambda type. In
other cases fragments of immunoglobulin or a totally different
protein (protein A) may be the source of the fibrils. A small amount
of muco-polysaccharide is usually present but this is probably
derived from the interstitial ground substance.

STAINING OF AMYLOID

1. Iodine and dilute sulphuric acid may produce blue colouration
    similar to that obtained with starch (Latin-amylum)
2. Congo-red—stains amyloid orange/red which under polarised
    light gives a green birefringence
3. Methyl violet—amyloid is rose pink
4. Thioflavine-T causes yellow fluorescence when viewed by
    ultraviolet light

SITES OF DEPOSITION

A. *General pattern*

Most cases show deposition in
1. Kidneys
2. Spleen
3. Liver

and frequently in
4. Intestine
5. Adrenals
6. Lymph nodes
7. Pancreas

This pattern reflects deposition of amyloid in relation to the reticulin of basement membranes beneath the endothelium of blood vessels or sinusoids (peri-reticulin deposition). A less typical pattern of involvement is found where the amyloid is deposited in relation to collagen fibres in the adventitia of blood vessels, the connective tissue of various organs, muscle sarcolemma, and neurolemma of peripheral nerves. This pericollagen pattern involves:
1. Heart
2. Lung
3. Gingiva
4. Tongue
5. Gastrointestinal tract

The atypical (pericollagen) pattern is the distribution usually found in primary amyloidosis and in that associated with multiple myeloma, but there is considerable overlap between these two basic patterns.

B. *Organ involvement*
1. Kidney—may be enlarged and pale
   Amyloid is deposited in:
   (i) Glomeruli (mesangium and basement membrane)
   (ii) Around basement membranes of tubules
   (iii) Blood vessels
   Results in:
   (i) Nephrotic syndrome
   (ii) Increased incidence of renal vein thrombosis
   (iii) Haematuria
   (iv) Nephrogenic diabetes insipidus
2. Spleen
   Deposited in:
   (i) Focal pattern in Malpighian bodies (sago spleen)
   (ii) Diffusely in the walls of sinusoids

3. Liver
   Deposited in:
   (i) The space of Disse between the sinusoid-lining cells and the liver cells
   (ii) Blood vessels
   Results in:
   (i) Pressure atrophy of liver cells which may in extreme cases lead to liver failure
   (ii) Portal hypertension, when involvement of central veins results in outflow obstruction (rare)
4. Heart
   Deposited in:
   (i) Subendocardial zone
   (ii) Interstitial connective tissue·
   Results in:
   (i) Cardiomegaly and failure
   (ii) Disturbances of rhythm
5. Adrenal gland
   Deposited in the zona glomerulosa and then advances centrally
   Results in:
   Addison's disease (rarely)
6. Gastrointestinal tract (from mouth to anus)
   Deposited in:
   (i) Walls of small blood vessels
   (ii) As plaques in the submucosa
   Results in:
   (i) Macroglossia
   (ii) Dysphagia resulting from oesophageal rigidity
   (iii) Malabsorption syndrome
   (iv) Diarrhoea
   (v) Protein-losing enteropathy
   (vi) Obstruction
   (vii) Ulceration
7. Skin
   (1) Primary amyloidosis
      a. Lichen amyloidosis
      b. Localised nodular amyloidosis
      c. Primary systematised amyloid sometimes shows nodular or papular skin lesions
   (ii) Secondary amyloidosis very rarely involves skin

THEORIES OF AMYLOID DEPOSITION

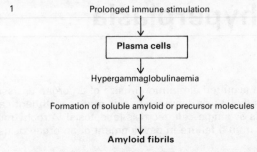

1   Prolonged immune stimulation

Plasma cells

Hypergammaglobulinaemia

Formation of soluble amyloid or precursor molecules

Amyloid fibrils

Deposited from the blood vessels into subendothelial 'spaces'

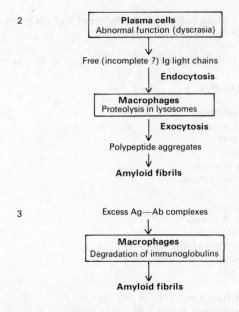

2   **Plasma cells**
         Abnormal function (dyscrasia)

Free (incomplete ?) Ig light chains

Endocytosis

Macrophages
Proteolysis in lysosomes

Exocytosis

Polypeptide aggregates

Amyloid fibrils

3   Excess Ag—Ab complexes

Macrophages
Degradation of immunoglobulins

Amyloid fibrils

FURTHER READING

Glenner, G.G. (1972) The discovery of the immunoglobulin origin of amyloid fibrils and its pathogenetic significance. *Acta Pathologica et Microbiologica Scandinavica,* Suppl. **233**, 114.

Stirling, G.A. (1975) Amyloidosis. *Recent Advances in Pathology,* 9, eds. Harrison, C.V. & Weinbren, K. p. 249. Edinburgh: Churchill Livingstone.

Atrophy, hypertrophy and hyperplasia

ATROPHY

Atrophy is the acquired diminution in size of an organ or tissue brought about by loss or decrease in size of its constituent cells. Loss of cells is by single-cell necrosis (apoptosis). Atrophy must be distinguished from a failure in development of an organ or tissue.

Hypoplasia is a partial failure of development whereby an organ does not attain the normal size, e.g. hypoplasia of one or both kidneys.

Agenesis is a complete failure of development e.g. congenital absence of one or both kidneys.

Atrophy can occur under physiological or pathological conditions:

A. Physiological atrophy
1. In the fetus
   - (i) Branchial clefts
   - (ii) Thyroglossal duct
   - (iii) Notochord
2. In the neonate
   - (i) Ductus arteriosus
   - (ii) Umbilical vessels
   - (iii) Urachus
3. Post adolescence
   - (i) Lymphoid tissue
     - a. Tonsils
     - b. Mesenteric lymph glands
     - c. Appendix
     - d. Thymus
4. In the adult
   - (i) Post-partum involution of the uterus
   - (ii) Post-lactational atrophy of the breasts
   - (iii) Post-menopausal atrophy of the uterus and ovaries

B. Pathological atrophy
  1. Localised atrophy
      (i)   Ischaemia, e.g. cerebral atrophy due to atherosclerosis
      (ii) Pressure
            a. Aortic aneurysm eroding bone
            b. Meningioma causing atrophy of overlying skull
            c. Hydronephrosis producing atrophy of the kidney
               parenchyma
      (iii) Disuse
            a. Local osteoporosis and muscular atrophy resulting
               from immobilisation
            b. Obstruction of a duct draining an exocrine gland
               leads to atrophy of the glandular elements, e.g.
               salivary gland
      (iv) Miscellaneous
            a. As part of muscular dystrophies
            b. Atrophy of the thyroid in myxoedema
            c. Testicular atrophy, in cirrhosis, oestrogen therapy,
               etc.
            d. Adrenal atrophy in idiopathic Addison's disease
            e. Gastric parietal-cell atrophy in pernicious anaemia
            f. Villous atrophy in coeliac disease
  2. Generalised atrophy results from:
      (i)   Simple starvation, severe malnutrition, malabsorption
            and malignant cachexia. There is:
            a. Muscle wasting
            b. Loss of adipose tissue
            c. 'Brown atrophy' of the heart
            d. Microsplanchnia
      (ii) Senility
      (iii) Hypopituitarism
      (iv) Osteoporosis—generalised atrophy of bone

HYPERTROPHY

Hypertrophy is the increase in size of an organ or tissue brought
about by an increase in *size* of its specialised cells. In a pure form,
hypertrophy is found only in muscle and is usually a response to an
increased demand for work. A further rare cause is the hypertrophy
of the tongue and heart seen in acromegaly resulting from
increased stimulation by growth hormone.
  1. Cardiac muscle
      (i)   Left ventricle (>1.5 cm average thickness)
            a. Systemic hypertension
            b. Aortic valvular disease
            c. Mitral incompetence
            d. High-output states such as severe anaemia,
               hypercapnia, thyrotoxicosis
            e. Hypertrophic cardiomyopathy

    (ii)   Right ventricle (>0.4 cm thickness)
        a. Chronic lung disease—cor pulmonale
        b. Mitral stenosis
        c. Secondary to left ventricular failure
        d. Congenital left to right shunts
        e. Pulmonary or tricuspid valvular lesions

2. Skeletal muscle—exercise
3. Smooth muscle
    (i)   Uterus—pregnancy
    (ii)   Arteries—hypertension (medial hypertrophy)
    (iii) Alimentary tract (usually proximal to an obstruction) e.g.
        a. Above an oesophageal stricture
        b. Proximal to an annular carcinoma of the colon
        also
        c. Idiopathic hypertrophic pyloric stenosis
    (iv) Urinary bladder (obstruction to outflow)
        a. Prostatic enlargement
        b. Urethral stricture
        c. Meatal stricture
        d. Severe phimosis
        e. Congenital bladder neck obstruction

Hypertrophy is recognised by *trabeculation* of the mucosal lining.

HYPERPLASIA

Hyperplasia is an increase in size of an organ or tissue brought about by an increase in *number* of its specialised cells. In many cases hyperplasia is associated with some degree of hypertrophy of individual cells.

1. *Endocrine glands*
    (i)   Adrenal cortex
        a. ACTH administration
        b. Basophil adenoma of the pituitary
        c. Idiopathic hyperplasia
        d. Congenital adrenal hyperplasia
    (ii)   Parathyroids
        a. Primary (idiopathic) hyperplasia
        b. Secondary to chronic renal failure
    (iii) Thyroid—primary thyrotoxicosis (Graves' disease)
    (iv) Pituitary
        a. Acidophil hyperplasia is an occasional cause of
           acromegaly
        b. Basophil hyperplasia—Cushing's syndrome
    (v)   Pancreatic islets
        Hyperplasia is seen in the babies of diabetic mothers

2. *Endocrine target organs*
   (i)   Breasts
      a. Physiological hyperplasia in pregnancy and lactation
      b. Pathological in cystic disease of the breast
   (ii) Endometrium
      Cystic hyperplasia in response to excessive oestrogen
      stimulation
   (iii) Prostate—benign nodular hyperplasia

3. *Skin*
   (i)   Prickle-cell hyperplasia (acanthosis) is seen in many skin
      diseases including
      a. Psoriasis (in the rete pegs)
      b. Chronic dermatitis
      c. Acanthosis nigricans
      d. Viral warts
   (ii) Pseudo-epitheliomatous hyperplasia is seen
      a. In association with chronic inflammation and
         granulation tissue
      b. Overlying dermal tumours such as granular-cell
         myoblastoma
      c. In kerato-acanthoma

4. *Lining epithelia*
   e.g. at the margins of healing ulcers in the stomach, duodenum
   or colon

5. *Bone marrow*
   Hyperplasia is most commonly seen where demand for red blood
   cells is increased by
   (i)   Haemolytic states
   (ii) Hypoxia

Metaplasia, dysplasia and carcinoma-in-situ

METAPLASIA

—is the transformation of one type of differentiated tissue into another type of fully differentiated tissue. Transformation within neoplastic tissue is referred to as 'tumour metaplasia'.

A. Epithelial
1. Squamous metaplasia
   - (i) From pseudo-stratified columnar ciliated epithelium
     - a. In the trachea and bronchi in chronic bronchitis, cigarette smokers, bronchiectasis
     - b. In nasal sinuses, (occasionally) in chronic sinusitis and in hypovitaminosis A
   - (ii) From simple columnar epithelium
     - a. Endometrium in senility
     - b. Gall-bladder in cholelithiasis
     - c. Prostatic ducts in ageing and oestrogen therapy
     - d. Endocervical mucosa and glands associated with cervical 'erosion'
   - (iii) From mesothelium of the pleura and peritoneum
2. Columnar metaplasia
   - (i) 'Pink-cell' or apocrine metaplasia seen in cystic disease of the breast
   - (ii) Intestinal metaplasia of the gastric mucosa in chronic atrophic gastritis
   - (iii) In mesothelium of peritoneum, pleura and synovium

B. Connective tissue
1. Osseous metaplasia
   - (i) In sites of dystrophic calcification
     - a. Scars
     - b. Old tuberculous lesions
     - c. Medial calcification of arteries
   - (ii) In muscle
     - a. Localised myositis ossificans
     - b. Post-traumatic
     - c. After tetanus
     - d. Paraplegia
   - (iii) In soft tissues
     - a. Tumoral calcinosis(?)
     - b. Progressive fibrodysplasia ossificans
     - c. Pseudo-hypoparathyroidism
     - d. Hereditary osteodystrophy (Albright's)
2. Myeloid metaplasia
   Development of haemopoietic tissue in the metaplastic bone

124

EPITHELIAL DYSPLASIA
—a disturbance of growth which is usually considered to be pre-malignant.
Dysplasia is evidenced by:
  (i)   Pleomorphism of cells (variation in size and shape)
  (ii)   Hyperchromatic nuclei and increased mitotic activity
  (iii) Loss of polarity (orientation) of cells
  (iv)   Disordered maturation
  (v)   No invasion
In columnar secretory epithelium there may be loss of mucin production, whilst squamous epithelium may show deep single-cell keratinisation (*dyskeratosis*).

Milder degrees of dysplasia may represent a reaction to underlying inflammation, whilst the most severe changes indicate a diagnosis of intra-epithelial carcinoma or *carcinoma-in-situ*.
Dysplasia and carcinoma-in-situ are found in the:
  (i)   Cervix (squamous epithelium)
  (ii)   Large-intestine complicating ulcerative colitis
  (iii) Gastric mucosa
  (iv)   Larynx, usually associated with keratosis
  (v)   Oro-pharynx and vulva, as 'leukoplakia'
  (vi)   Skin—senile or solar keratosis
  (vii) Breast—severe epitheliosis, intra-duct and intra-lobular carcinoma

Special forms of carcinoma-in-situ
  (i)   Paget's disease of the skin usually associated with an underlying adenocarcinoma and characterised by the presence of large clear intra-epidermal cells—Paget cells. In some cases direct spread to the skin cannot be excluded.
         Sites:
         a. Nipple
         b. Anus
         c. Vulva
         d. Axilla
  (ii)   Bowen's disease of the skin (intra-epidermal carcinoma)
  (iii) Erythroplasia of Queyrat—intra-epidermal carcinoma occurring on the glans penis, the vulva, or the oral mucosa

EXFOLIATIVE CYTOLOGY
Surface cells are constantly desquamated from epithelial and mesothelial linings and can be examined in secretions or in centrifuged deposits of smears of effusions, urine, etc. Where the epithelium is directly accessible a scraping of the surface cells provides better material for cytological examination.

Uses of exfoliative cytology

1. Cancer detection in suspected cases
2. Cytological screening
3. Follow-up after treatment
4. Hormonal cytology
5. Nuclear sexing
6. Viral inclusion disease
7. Assessment of fetal maturity

1. *Cancer detection*
    (i)   Cervix—cervical smears
    (ii)   Bladder—urine deposits
    (iii)   Bronchus—sputum or brushings via endoscope
    (iv)   Serous effusions—aspirate
    (v)   Stomach—washings or brushings
    (vi)   Breast—aspiration of cyst fluid or nipple discharge

2. *Cytological screening*
    (i)   Urine from dye or rubber-workers (increased incidence of urothelial carcinoma)
    (ii)   Cervical smears from 'normal' women

3. *Follow-up*
    (i)   Post-irradiation, especially for carcinoma of the bladder and cervix
    (ii)   Post-resection—bladder tumour

4. *Hormonal cytology*
—scrapings from upper 1/3 of vagina or aspiration from the posterior fornix.
Oestrogens have a keratinising effect whereas progestogens tend to arrest maturation at the intermediate stage ('boat-cells'). Such assessment is useful in the investigation of amenorrhoea and oestrogen-producing tumours.

5. *Nuclear sexing*
—scrapings of buccal mucosa or squamous cells from the skin
A peripheral dot of chromatin can be found in the nuclei of cells from females (XX) and is termed the sex-chromatin or Barr body. This is considered to be an inactive X-chromosome and the number of Barr bodies found is one less than the number of X-chromosomes in that nucleus. Thus the normal male (XY) does not exhibit a Barr body, whilst 'super-females' (XXX) possess two Barr bodies per nucleus

6. *Viral inclusion disease*
Cytomegalic inclusion infection may be diagnosed by finding the characteristic inclusions in cells obtained from urine

7. *Assessment of fetal maturity*

Aspirates of amniotic fluid are examined for the presence of laguno hairs and desquamated cells laden with fat droplets. If the fluid contains 20% or more of such cells the fetus is 36 weeks or more

FURTHER READING

Bate, J.G. (1969) Evaluation of cervical cytology. *British Journal of Hospital Medicine,* **2,** 952.

Coleman, D.V. (1969) The clinical application of exfoliative cytology. *British Journal of Hospital Medicine,* **2,** 1499.

Hughes, H.E. & Dodds, T.C. (1968) *Handbook of Diagnositc Cytology.* Edinburgh: E. & S. Livingstone.

Phillips, A.J. (Ed.) (1974) *Cancer Detection.* International Union against Cancer Monograph, 4. New York: Springer Verlag.

Neoplasia

Tumours are usually divided on the basis of their behaviour into two main groups, benign and malignant.

The principal points of distinction between the two groups are:

	Benign	Malignant
Mode of growth	Expansive	Infiltrative and expansive
	Circumscribed	Poorly-defined margins
	Encapsulated	
Rate of growth	Slow and may cease	Rapid
Microscopic structure	Well-differentiated (i.e. closely resembles tissue of origin)	Varying degrees of differentiation
	Cells—regular	Cellular pleomorphism (variation in size and shape)
	Absent or scanty mitotic figures	Increased mitoses
Metastases	Absent	Frequently present
Clinical effects	Mechanical or hormonal	Mechanical, hormonal, destructive, systemic effects
Outcome	Rarely fatal	Usually fatal

These are general points to which there are many exceptions. Some tumours exhibit an intermediate type of behaviour and cannot be allocated to either category, e.g. giant-cell tumour of bone

Tumours are currently classified according to their behaviour and tissue of origin.

Tissue of origin	Benign	Malignant
Epithelium		
Surface or lining epithelium	Papilloma	Carcinoma
Secretory epithelium (glandular or lining)	Adenoma	Adenocarcinoma
Connective Tissue		
Fibrous tissue	Fibroma	Fibrosarcoma
Fat	Lipoma	Liposarcoma
Bone	Osteoma	Osteosarcoma (osteo genic sarcoma)
Cartilage	Chondroma	Chondrosarcoma
Smooth muscle	Leiomyoma	Leiomyosarcoma
Striated muscle	Rhabdomyoma	Rhabdomyosarcoma
Blood vessels	Haemangioma	Angiosarcoma
Lymphoid tissue		Malignant lymphoma
Nervous system		Astrocytoma, Oligodendroglioma and Ependymoma
Trophoblast	Hydatidiform mole	Chorion carcinoma
Embryonic tissue		
Totipotent cells	Benign teratoma	Malignant teratoma
Pluripotent cells		Nephroblastoma Hepatoblastoma
Unipotent cells		Medulloblastoma (brain) Retinoblastoma
	Ganglioneuroma	Neuroblastoma (sympathetic nerve)

COMPLICATIONS OF BENIGN TUMOURS
1. Pressure effects
    (i) Meningioma compressing brain or spinal-cord
    (ii) Uterine leiomyoma (fibroid) compressing bladder or rectum
2. Obstruction
    (i) Bronchial obstruction due to an adenoma
    (ii) Blockage of the mitral valve by an atrial myxoma
    (iii) CSF obstruction by an ependymoma
3. Ulceration and haemorrhage
    (i) Leiomyoma of the stomach wall

      (ii)   Haemorrhage into an ovarian tumour or leiomyoma of the uterus

4. Infarction, e.g. pedunculated fibroid
5. Infection, e.g. transitional cell papilloma of bladder
6. Rupture of cystic neoplasms, e.g. mucin-secreting cystadeno-carcinoma of the ovary producing myxoma peritonii
7. Hormone production
    (i) Islet-cell tumour of the pancreas producing insulin or gastrin
    (ii) Phaeochromocytoma
    (iii) Adrenal cortical adenoma giving rise to
        a. Cushing's syndrome
        b. Conn's syndrome
    (iv) Pituitary adenoma
        a. Acromegaly
        b. Cushing's syndrome
    (v) Parathyroid adenoma
8. Malignant change
    e.g. Adenomatous polyp of large intestine giving rise to adenocarcinoma, as occurs in familial polyposis

TERATOMA

A teratoma is 'a true tumour composed of multiple tissues foreign to the part in which it arises' (Willis).

There are two main theories of origin:

1. A nest of totipotent cells, usually from the primitive streak, escapes from the effects of primary organisers during embryonic development, and later develops into a bizarre admixture of tissues
2. Teratomas originate by neoplastic change in germ cells (which may have arrested in their migration from the yolk sac wall) possibly brought about by mutation of the growth-controlling locus in these cells

Sites
1. Ovary (usually benign)
2. Testis (usually malignant)
3. Anterior mediastinum
4. Presacral
5. Retroperitoneal
6. Intrapericardial
7. Base of skull and nasopharynx
8. Intracranial, including pineal
9. Neck—usually within the thyroid gland

HAMARTOMA

A hamartoma is a tumour-like malformation composed of a haphazard arrangement of tissues appropriate to the particular part of the body in which it is found. The distinction between a hamartoma and a benign tumour can be very difficult, and occasionally malignant tumours develop from such malformations.

Examples

1. *Respiratory system*
    (i) Pulmonary hamartoma composed principally of mature cartilage but including columnar or cuboidal epithelium and fibrous tissue (sometimes termed adenochondroma)

2. *Vascular system*
    (i) Capillary haemangioma of skin
    (ii) Cavernous haemangioma
    (iii) Lymphangioma, e.g. cystic 'hygroma' of infancy

3. *Skin*
    (i) Derived from altered epidermal melanocytes
        a. Junctional naevus
        b. Compound naevus
        c. Intral-dermal naevus
    (ii) Derived from altered melanocytes arrested in their migration through the dermis
        a. Blue naevus
        b. Mongolian blue spot
        c. Oculodermal melanosis

4. *Intestine*
    e.g. Peutz-Jehger's polyps in the small intestine associated with circumoral pigmentation

5. *Nervous system*
    e.g. Neurofibromatosis

6. *Skeletal system*
    e.g. Solitary or multiple exostoses

7. *Multi-system involvement*
    Tuberous sclerosis
    (i) Skin papules—'Adenoma sebaceum'
    (ii) Gliomas
    (iii) Rhabdomyomas in the heart
    (iv) Angiolipomyoma in the kidney (These can occur without other stigmata of tuberous sclerosis)

GROWTH AND SPREAD OF TUMOURS

The most important characteristics of tumours are their capacity for:
A.   Unco-ordinated growth—common to all tumours
B.   Invasion—the fundamental property of malignant tumours

A. *Tumour growth* is the resultant of:
1.   Mitotic activity of the tumour cells
2.   Death of cells by:
     (i)   Apoptosis
     (ii) Infarction

It progresses in two ways:
1.   *Expansive growth.* Purely expansive growth is a feature of many benign tumours and produces a circumscribed, encapsulated neoplasm, e.g. fibroadenoma of the breast
2.   *Infiltrative growth* is usually a reflection of invasion and can be recognised around the margins of an otherwise expansile malignant epithelial tumour. However, infiltration is seen around the margins of some benign connective tissue tumours, e.g. dermato-fibroma, and is less helpful in distinguishing benign from malignant.

B. *Invasion*
Direct spread of tumour in continuity occurs along the following:
1.   Microscopic tissue spaces (interstitial spread)
2.   Lymphatic permeation, as a continuous cord of tumour cells
3.   Veins and capillary blood vessels, e.g. renal carcinoma along the renal vein
4.   Coelomic cavities, e.g. pleural spread of lung cancer
5.   Cerebrospinal spaces, e.g. malignant gliomas
6.   Epithelial cavities, e.g. uterine tumours spreading along the Fallopian tubes

The mechanisms underlying the invasive properties of malignant cells are not known. The following factors have been suggested as possible explanations.

1. *Progressive multiplication and transplantability*
Malignant cells can be grown more easily than normal cells *in vitro* where they undergo rapid proliferation. It is suggested that *in vivo* progressive multiplication and expansive growth raise intra-tumour tissue pressure which forces cells along lines of cleavage into surrounding tissues. Some rapidly proliferating tumours are entirely benign, however, and show no tendency to invade.

2. *Motility and loss of adhesiveness*
Malignant cells display greater motility and less adhesion *in vitro* than normal epithelial cells.

Increased motility may be related to a higher content of contractile proteins.

Loss of adhesiveness may result from:

    (i)   Failure to form intercellular junctions (desmosomes)

    (ii)   Lack of calcium at the cell surface. Calcium ions form an anionic bond between cells by neutralising the mutually repellant negative groups on their surfaces. Tumour tissue contains less calcium than normal and there is therefore a higher repellent negative charge on the cells tending to prevent cell adhesion

3. Loss of contact inhibition

When normal cells which are proliferating and spreading come into contact a 'cut-out' mechanism operates and mitosis and movement ceases. Malignant cells show a loss of such 'contact inhibition' and proliferation persists. Contact inhibition may be related to *chalone* synthesis.

Chalones are short-lived, water-soluble glycoproteins or polypeptides which inhibit mitosis. They are locally-produced and tissue specific. The failure of malignant cells to show the normal inhibition of mitosis on contact may be due to:

    (i)   Local failure of chalone production

    (ii)   Abnormal production of anti-chalones

    (iii) Lack of responsiveness to chalones by tumour cells

4. Production of enzymes

Tumour cells produce enzymes, such as hyaluronidase and aminopeptidase, which may lyse or destroy normal cells or stroma and facilitate invasion.

5. Fibrin production

Fibrin is deposited around the growing margins of many tumours. The organisation of this deposit may lead to the formation of blood vessels, lymphatics and stroma, bringing nutrition to the tumour and encouraging its growth. On the other hand, the fibrin deposit may be a host reaction tending to limit the growth of the tumour. Its role in tumour spread is therefore doubtful.

METASTASIS

Denotes successful growth of tumour in the body at a site distant from its primary location.

Detached tumour cells take the following paths:

1. Lymphatics
2. Blood vessels
3. Coelomic spaces
4. Cerebrospinal spaces
5. Epithelial cavities

1. *Lymphatic spread* is most commonly associated with carcinomas, but is frequently seen with malignant melanoma and malignant teratoma of the testis.

Results of lymph node involvement:
- (i)   Compression of neighbouring structures e.g. superior vena cava syndrome
- (ii) Invasion of adjacent tissues:
    - a. veins
    - b. trachea, skin, etc.
- (iii) Further dissemination by diversion of lymph flow
- (iv) Lymphoedema of limb or scrotum

2. *Blood spread* occurs typically with sarcomas and as a later feature of spread from carcinomas. There are three continuous phases:
- (i)   The invasion of blood vessels by tumour cells
    Mechanism (?)
    - a. Increased tissue pressure in the tumour forcing cells into vascular lumina
    - b. Imperfect endothelial lining of tumour blood vessels allowing direct access by tumour cells (especially in sarcomas)
    - c. Loss of cell-to-cell adhesiveness
- (ii) The transport of tumour cells by established vascular pathways. The presence of circulating tumour cells does not inevitably lead to metastases, however
- (iii) The lodgement, attachment, and growth of tumour cells at the distant site

The arrest of circulating tumour cells is not a result of non-specific mechanical trapping, but probably is determined by the cell surface properties of the tumour cell. The variation in these surface properties and their differing affinity for arrest may explain the organ specificity of metastatic tumour spread.

Examples of organ specificity
- a. Carcinoma of the breast, thyroid, kidney, lung and prostate frequently metastasise to bone
- b. Carcinoma of the bronchus often involves the liver and adrenals
- c. Seminoma (testis) spreads to the lung
- d. Sarcomas spread principally to the lung but also to liver and brain

3. *Coelomic spaces*
Examples
- (i)   Spread from a gastric or intestinal primary to the ovaries (Krukenberg tumours)
- (ii) Pleural spread of lung and breast cancer

4. *Cerebrospinal spaces*
Primary tumours of the CNS may spread via the subarachnoid space

or the ventricular system and give rise to seedlings distant from their origin.

5. Epithelial cavities
Apart from implantation of desquamated tumour cells from an intestinal carcinoma into anastomosis sites during surgical removal, this mode of spread is rare.

AETIOLOGY OF TUMOURS
The following factors are considered to be important in oncogenesis:
A. Physical
B. Chemical
C. Viral
D. Hormonal
E. Immunological

A. Physical
1. Solar radiation—squamous carcinoma of the skin
2. X-irradiation
   (i) Skin cancer
   (ii) Leukaemia
3. Radio-active substances
   (i) Lung cancer due to radon (Schneeburg miners)
   (ii) Osteogenic sarcoma following ingestion of radium, strontium, mesothorium (luminous paint)
4. Heat (?)—Changri cancer of the abdominal wall (charcoal braziers tied around abdomen by Kashmiri)

B. Chemical
Of largely historical interest, early examples of chemical carcinogenesis are:
1. Carcinoma of the scrotum in chimney-sweeps
2. Cancer of the hands and arms in shale-oil workers
3. Cancer of the skin and lung after long-term exposure to arsenic (still seen occasionally)
Present day examples are:
4. Carcinoma of the lung
   (i) Tobacco smoke
   (ii) Asbestos
   (iii) Chromate smelting
5. Carcinoma of the bladder
   (i) Aniline dye production
   (ii) Rubber manufacture
6. Carcinoma of the nasal sinuses in wood-workers
7. Carcinoma of the skin in tar-workers

Experimental carcinogenesis
Most, if not all, chemical carcinogens undergo some metabolic conversion to form active alkylating or arylating products which bind

to DNA, RNA and protein. These active products are termed the *proximate carcinogens* and can modify the genome of the cell by:
1. Direct action on DNA
2. Modification of tRNA followed by the production of mutant DNA by the reverse transcriptase mechanism

Chemical carcinogens
1. Locally-acting chemical carcinogens,
   e.g. polycyclic aromatic hydrocarbons such as 3:4 benzpyrene, 3:methylcholanthrene
   These are 'strong' carcinogens characterised by:
   (i) Action at the site of administration
   (ii) Most tissues will respond
   (iii) High tumour yield
2. Remotely-acting carcinogens
   e.g. *N*-methyl-4-aminoazobenzene (MAB) produces liver tumours after oral administration because the liver is the site of its metabolic conversion to the carcinogenic *N*-hydroxy derivative. 2-Acetylaminofluorene produces tumours in many different organs after oral administration

Biology of carcinogenesis
1. The effects of carcinogens are dose-dependent, additive, and irreversible.
2. Carcinogenesis occurs after a variable latent period during which a series of modifications occurs converting a normal cell, through successive generations, into a cancer cell. Such modifications are accelerated and enhanced by cell proliferation, and chemicals promoting the change from a modified to malignant cell may not be carcinogenic themselves, e.g. Croton oil

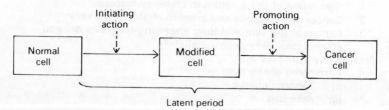

3. Carcinogenesis is influenced by other biological factors including:
   (i) Age
   (ii) Sex
   (iii) Diet
   (iv) Hormones
   (v) Chronic inflammation

C. Hormonal
Whilst it is well known that hormones can greatly modify the production and growth of tumours, their role in the causation of tumours is less clear. It may well be that hormones act as promoters of malignant change already initiated by some other factor such as virus or chemicals.

Examples
1. Oestrogens
   (i)   In mice oestrogens promote the development of mammary cancer which has been initiated by the Bittner virus
   (ii) Administration of artifical oestrogens to trans-sexual men has resulted in a few cases of mammary carcinoma
   (iii) Breast carcinoma in women may undergo regression after adrenalectomy and oophorectomy
   (iv) Hyperoestrogenism, for example due to a granulosa cell tumour of the ovary, may give rise to endometrial carcinoma
2. Trophic hormones
   (i)   Gonadotrophins will bring about proliferation and in some cases malignant change in the ovaries of experimental animals which have been transplanted into the spleen. In this site the oestrogens released by the ovary are inactivated by the liver and there is reduced feed-back to the pituitary which responds by excessive production of gonadotrophins
   (ii) Excess TSH and ACTH levels may bring about tumour formation in the corresponding target organs in experimental animals

D. Viral
Many animal tumours are now attributable to oncogenic viruses, e.g. leukaemia and sarcoma in chickens, but only a few human neoplasms have been associated with viruses and there are no malignant tumours in which a causal relationship has been established.
1. Warts (squamous papillomata) are caused by a papova virus
2. Burkitt's lymphoma has some relationship with the herpes-type Epstein-Barr (EB) virus. It is possible that infection by EB virus in an individual with a normal immune system results in infectious mononucleosis (glandular fever) whereas infection in an individual, usually a child, with immuno-deficiency or an immune system altered by chronic malaria, results in a malignant lymphoma
3. Naso-pharyngeal carcinoma is also associated with raised anti-bodies to the EB virus
4. Virions similar to the Bittner virus have been identified in milk from women with a close family history of breast carcinoma and in breast cancer cells
5. A higher incidence of antibodies to herpes simplex virus type 2 is found in women with carcinoma of the cervix

Mechanism
1. DNA viruses are incorporated into the cell genome and may bring about neoplastic transformation
2. RNA viruses may modify the host cell DNA by an RNA-directed DNA polymerase—the reverse transcriptase pathway.

E. Immunological

The immunological theories of oncogenesis depend upon some breakdown of the normal capacity to recognise neoplastic cells as 'foreign' and to react against them. This ability to recognise mutant cells is termed 'immunological surveillance'. The existence of immunological surveillance presumes that there are antigenic differences between normal and neoplastic cells. Evidence for the development of tumour antigens and immune reactions to them has been drawn from animals and humans.

Evidence in animals
1. Syngeneic animals can reject transplanted tumour if previously immunised against it (e.g. with irradiated tumour cells)
2. The presence of circulating antibodies cytotoxic to tumour cells *in vitro* has been demonstrated in viral-induced animal leukaemias
3. Immune lymphocytes produced in one animal will cause regression of chemically-induced tumours when injected into syngeneic animals
4. After a primary solid tumour has been removed from an animal, it is more difficult to re-establish the tumour and a larger inoculum must be given
5. Animals rendered immunodeficient by neonatal thymectomy or made tolerant to tumour antigens are more susceptible to oncogenesis

Evidence in man
1. Circulating antibodies to tumour antigens have been demonstrated in malignant melanoma, neuroblastoma, Burkitt's lymphoma and nasopharyngeal carcinoma (which cross-react with EB virus), osteogenic sarcoma, etc.
2. Cell-mediated immunity can be demonstrated to tumour specific antigens by macrophage migration inhibition, etc.
3. Histological evidence.
    With certain tumours, those that have a prominent lymphocytic stromal infiltrate ('host reaction') have a better prognosis

4. Immunodeficiency or suppression is associated with an increased incidence of tumours
5. Tumour cells which have been inadvertently transplanted into the recipients of renal homografts taken from cancer patients have grown successfully because of immunosuppression of the host.

The following may have an immunological basis:

6. Spontaneous regression
7. Dramatic response after small doses of chemotherapy, e.g. in Burkitt's lymphoma and chorioncarcinoma
8. Removal of a primary tumour may be followed by regression of secondaries
9. Long-standing relapses after presumed 'dormancy' of cancer cells

Development of tumour antigens
Alteration of the genome by the oncogenic agent may lead to the formation of new antigens at the cell surface. These might not respond to humoral (chalone) and contact stimuli appropriately and react by excessive proliferation.

(i)   Virus alteration results in a new surface antigen which is characteristic of the infecting virus and common to all tumours produced by that virus
(ii) Chemical carcinogens also induce new surface antigens but these differ from tumour to tumour (idiotypic)

Failure of the immune response may be due to:

1. Tumours not antigenic
2. Host's immune system inefficient
    (i)   Increasing age
    (ii)   Genetically-determined
        a. Specific immune failure
        b. General immunodeficiency states
        (? related to HLA status)
    (iii) Tolerance
        a. Oncogenic virus transmitted vertically or present from birth
        b. High dose suppression by the tumour itself
    (iv)   Iatrogenic immunosuppression
    (v)   Blocking of cytotoxic effects on the tumour cells by
        a. Free tumour antigen
        b. Soluble immune complexes
        c. Anti-IgG (directed against anti-tumour antibodies)

NON-METASTATIC EFFECTS OF TUMOURS

A. Skin markers of malignancy
1. Acanthosis nigricans
    almost always associated with carcinoma—75%
    adenocarcinoma
2. Dermatomyositis
    about 15% of cases associated with malignancy
3. Dermatitis herpetiformis
    with hydatidiform mole,
        chorioncarcinoma
4. Exfoliative dermatitis
    with lymphomas and leukaemias
5. Erythema gyratum repens
    with carcinoma of the bronchus
6. Pigmentation
    in carcinomatosis
7. Pruritis
    in lymphomas and some carcinomas
8. Herpes zoster
    in Hodgkin's and lymphomas
9. Bullous pemphigoid (?)
10. Acquired ichthyosis
    in lymphomas
11. Fixed L-E like eruptions
12 Hypertrichosis
    (facial lanugo)

B. Neuromuscular effects
1. Myopathy
    with various carcinomas and lymphomas
2. Myasthenic syndrome
    with intrathoracic tumours usually oat-cell carcinoma of
    bronchus
3. Mixed neuropathy (sensory and motor)
    with many types of carcinoma, e.g. bronchus, stomach,
    breast, together with lymphomas and myeloma
4. Sensory neuropathy
    a rare complication of carcinoma of the bronchus
5. Autonomic neuropathy
6. Dementia or psychosis
7. Cerebellar degeneration
    with carcinoma of bronchus, breast, ovary and lymphomas
8. Brain stem degeneration
    may accompany some other neuromuscular lesion
9. Progressive multifocal leucoencephalopathy caused by papova
    virus
    very rare; association with lymphoma

C. Haematological effects

1. Thrombotic disorders
    (i)   Venous thrombosis
          especially carcinoma of the pancreas and mucin-producing carcinomas
    (ii) Non-bacterial thrombotic endocarditis
    (iii) Disseminated intravascular coagulation—prostate, bronchus, stomach, pancreas
    (iv) Microangiopathic haemolytic anaemia, usually advanced carcinoma of stomach, pancreas, colon, lung and breast
2. Miscellaneous
    (i)   Normocytic normochromic anaemia
    (ii) Autoimmune haemolytic anaemia
          Hodgkin's disease, lymphomas, thymoma
    (iii) Sideroblastic anaemia
    (iv) Thrombocytopenia
    (v)   Red cell aplasia associated with thymoma
    (vi) Polycythaemia with renal carcinoma, etc.

D. Hormonal effects—

due to inappropriate production by tumour cells

1. Cushing's syndrome (ACTH production)
    associated with oat-cell carcinoma of the bronchus, thymoma, carcinoid tumours, medullary carcinoma of the thyroid
2. Hyponatraemia—(ADH-like substance)
    oat cell carcinoma
3. Hypoglycaemia
    mesothelioma, liver cell carcinoma, adrenal cortical carcinoma
4. Hypercalcaemia (Calcitonin; prostaglandins; parathormone)
    with squamous carcinoma of the bronchus and cervix and renal carcinoma, lymphomas, breast carcinoma
5. Polycythaemia (erythropoietin production)
    from renal carcinoma and occasional cases of uterine leiomyoma, liver carcinoma, cerebellar haemangioblastoma, nephroblastoma
6. Carcinoid syndrome (5 H-T)
    oat-cell carcinoma, medullary carcinoma of the thyroid
7. Gynaecomastia
    with anaplastic or squamous carcinomas of bronchus
8. Hypertension (excess renin production)
    from nephroblastoma
9. Hyperthyroidism
    (i)   Hydatidiform mole and chorioncarcinoma
    (ii) Orchioblastoma
    (iii) Malignant teratoma trophoblastic of testis
10. Pigmentation (melanocyte stimulating hormone—MSH) from oat-cell carcinoma of bronchus

MALIGNANT TUMOURS OF CHILDHOOD

1. Leukaemia
   about 80% are acute lymphatic leukaemia
2. Lymphoma
   (i)   Non-Hodgkin's lymphoma including Burkitt's lymphoma
   (ii) Hodgkin's disease
3. Glioma
   (i)   Medulloblastoma (cerebellum)
   (ii) Astrocytoma, frequently sub-tentorial
   (iii) Ependymoma
4. Neuroblastoma
   From sympathetic ganglia and adrenal medulla
   Some mature into ganglioneuroma
5. Nephroblastoma
   Composed of tubules and immature glomeruli in a
   mesenchymal stroma which may contain striated muscle, fat,
   cartilage and bone
6. Hepatoblastoma
7. Orchioblastoma (testis)
8. Embryonal sarcomas
   Composed of primitive loose connective tissue which often
   contains striated muscle fibres (sarcoma botryoides)
   Sites:
   Female—vagina, urethra, trigone of the bladder
   Male—urethra, bladder, prostate
9. Osteogenic sarcoma
   Most commonly at the lower end of the femur, then the
   upper part of the tibia

FURTHER READING

Ambrose, E.J. & Roe, F.J.C. (Eds.) (1975) *Biology of Cancer,* 2nd
   edn. New York: Ellis Harwood Ltd.
Currie, G.A. (1974) Cancer and the immune response. *Current
   Topics in Immunology,* 2. London: Arnold.
Journal of Clinical Pathology, (1976) Malignancy in childhood:
   Symposium. *Journal of Clinical Pathology,* **29,** 1016.
Ratcliffe, J.G. & Rees, L.H. (1974) Clinical manifestations of ectopic
   hormone production. *British Journal of Hospital Medicine,* **11,**
   685.
Symington, T. & Carter, R.L. (Eds.) (1976) *Scientific Foundations of
   Oncology.* London: Heinemann.
Willis, R.A. (1973) *The Spread of Tumours in the Human Body,* 3rd.
   edn. London: Butterworth.

Biological effects of radiation

TYPES OF RADIATION
1. *X-Rays* are machine-generated electro-magnetic radiations of zero mass and charge
2. *γ-Rays* are similar to X-rays but are generated by the spontaneous decay of radio-active isotopes
3. *α-Particles* have a mass of 4 and a positive charge of 2 equivalent to a helium nucleus. They are produced by the nuclear reactions of high-energy electromagnetic radiation and the decay of radio-active elements, such as radium and uranium
4. *ß-Particles* are electrons having negligible mass and one negative charge, which in medical usage are produced by decay of certain isotopes

MECHANISMS OF ACTION
1. Direct action
   One mode of action may be a direct ionisation of part of a molecule by the absorbed energy.
2. Indirect action
   A more likely explanation is that highly reactive free radicals, such as uncharged hydrogen atoms or OH^0 radicals, are formed which subsequently attack intracellular macro-molecules causing cell injury.

CELLULAR EFFECTS
1. Very high dosage leads to rapid cell death
2. Lower doses by affecting DNA synthesis reduce mitotic activity
3. Chromosome abnormalities may appear after cell division

TISSUE EFFECTS
1. Skin, with increasing dosage
   (i) Erythema
   (ii) Abnormalities in pigmentation
   (iii) Hyperkeratosis
   (iv) Loss of skin appendages
   (v) Epidermal atrophy
   (vi) Dermal fibrosis
   (vii) Ulceration

2. Haemopoietic system
    (i)   Transient pancytopenia
    (ii)   Aplastic anaemia
    (iii) Leukaemic change
3. Testis
    (i)   Tubular atrophy and hyalinisation
    (ii)   Loss of spermatogonia
4. Ovary
    (i)   Destruction of follicles
    (ii)   Cessation of menstruation
5. Lungs
    (i)   Pulmonary congestion and oedema
    (ii)   'Hyaline membrane' reaction
    (iii) Interstitial fibrosis
    (iv)   Bronchial carcinoma following inhalation of radio-active
           substances, e.g. miners of Schneeberg (pitchblende)
6. Kidneys
    (i)   Glomerular fibrosis
    (ii)   Vascular sclerosis
    These changes may produce malignant hypertension
7. Gastrointestinal tract
    (i)   Mucosal oedema and ulceration
    (ii)   Vascular hyalinisation
    (iii) Submucosal fibrosis
    (iv)   Glandular atrophy
    (v)   Fibrosis of the muscularis propria
    (vi)   Stricture formation
8. Liver
    (i)   Diffuse fibrosis
    (ii)   Veno-occlusive disease
9. Bone
    (i)   'Radionecrosis'
    (ii)   Osteogenic sarcoma from radium and mesothorium
10. Nervous system
    (i)   White matter oedema
    (ii)   Astrocyte hypertrophy and hyperplasia
    (iii) Vascular hyalinisation
    (iv)   Microcalcification
    (v)   Necrosis probably mediated by small vessel fibrosis

WHOLE BODY IRRADIATION

With increasing dosage the effects can be grouped under three main syndromes:

1. Haemopoietic syndrome (100 rads +)
   (i)   Lymphopenia
   (ii) Granulocytopenia
   (iii) Thrombocytopenia
   Death may result from infection or haemorrhage.
2. Gastrointestinal syndrome (500 – 2000 rads)
   (i) Anorexia, nausea, vomiting
   (ii) Severe diarrhoea
   Death is due to fluid loss or electrolyte imbalance
3. Cerebral syndrome (above 2000 – 5000 rads)
   (i) Nausea, vomiting
   (ii) Tremors and convulsions
   Leading to death within hours or a day or two

If the patient survives the acute phase then there are a number of possible late effects:

1. Marrow aplasia
2. Cataracts
3. Developmental abnormalities in the fetus
4. Leukaemia, skin cancer, or cancer in other organs such as thyroid, bone, larynx, etc.
5. General effects—premature ageing
6. Pneumonitis; nephritis; myocarditis and pericarditis

SENSITIVITY OF TUMOURS TO IRRADIATION

The following factors are important:

1. Tissue of origin
2. Degree of differentiation, usually inversely proportional to the sensitivity
3. Mitotic activity, directly proportional to the sensitivity
4. Vascularity of the stroma and general blood supply, which is related to 5
5. Hypoxia reduces the sensitivity of tumours to radiation, conversely hyperbaric oxygen has been used to enhance radiotherapy
6. Recurrent tumours are insensitive as they are probably derived from the most radioresistant cells of the primary neoplasm.

FURTHER READING

Cancer (1976) Radiation therapy. Conference supplement. *Cancer,* **37**, 1090-1176.

Watkins, D.K. (1975) Lysosomes and radiation injury. *Lysosomes in Biology and Pathology* 4, eds. Dingle, J.T. & Dean, R.T. p. 147. London: North Holland.

Alimentary system

SALIVARY GLANDS

A. Congenital
1. Agenesis of one or more glands
2. Atresia of a duct

B. Acute inflammation
1. Acute suppurative sialadenitis
2. Mumps
3. Cytomegalic inclusion disease

C. Chronic inflammation
1. Non-specific, usually in association with calculi
2. Sjogren's syndrome
   - (i) Keratoconjunctivitis sicca
   - (ii) Xerostomia
   - (iii) Rheumatoid arthritis
   - (iv) Enlargement of salivary glands
3. Sarcoidosis
4. Tuberculosis
5. Actinomycosis
6. Syphilis
7. Mikulicz's disease (benign lymphoepithelial lesion)

D. Mechanical disorders
1. Mucocele resulting from rupture of a duct
2. Ranula results from obstruction of a sublingual gland
3. Obstruction by calculus—sialolithiasis

E. Benign tumours
1. Pleomorphic adenoma (mixed parotid tumour)
2. Papillary cystadenoma lymphomatosum (Warthin's tumour)
3. Monomorphic adenoma

F. Malignant tumours
1. Mucoepidermoid carcinoma
2. Adenoid cystic carcinoma (cylindroma)
3. Carcinoma arising from a pleomorphic adenoma
4. Adenocarcinoma

146

MOUTH AND PHARYNX

A. Congenital
1. Cleft lip and palate
2. Microstomia and macrostomia
3. Microglossia and macroglossia
4. Median rhomboid glossitis
5. 'Bifid' and 'scrotal' tongue

B. Acute inflammation
1. Non-specific gingivitis
2. Vincent's infection (acute necrotising ulcerative gingivitis)
3. Aphthous stomatitis
4. Herpetic gingivo-stomatitis
5. Moniliasis (thrush)
6. Cancrum oris (noma)

C. Chronic inflammation
1. Chronic desquamative gingivitis
2. Tuberculosis
3. Actinomycosis
4. Syphilis
   (i) Primary—chancre
   (ii) Secondary
       a. Mucous patches
       b. Snail-track ulcers
   (iii) Tertiary
       a. Localised gummata
       b. Diffuse involvement of the tongue
       c. Secondary leukoplakia

D. Benign tumours and tumour-like conditions
1. 'Congenital epulis'
2. Giant-cell epulis (probably reactive)
3. Angiomatous 'tumour' of pregnancy (reactive)
4. Fibroma
5. Haemangioma
6. Squamous papilloma
7. Lymphangioma
8. Granular-cell myoblastoma

E. Leukoplakia
Aetiology
   (i) Poor dental hygiene
   (ii) Smoking
   (iii) Trauma from rough teeth
   (iv) Syphilis
Microscopic appearances
   (i) Hyperplasia of squamous epithelium
   (ii) Hyperkeratosis
   (iii) Dysplasia (may be absent)
   (iv) Chronic inflammatory reaction

F. Malignant tumours
1. Squamous carcinoma
2. Adenocarcinoma (mucous/salivary glands)
3. Intermediate or 'transitional-cell' carcinoma (pharynx)
4. Undifferentiated carcinoma with lymphoid stroma—
   'lymphoepithelioma' (nasopharynx)
5. Malignant melanoma
6. Fibrosarcoma
7. Lymphoma (tonsils)

OESOPHAGUS
A. Congenital
1. Agenesis (extremely rare)
2. Atresia, usually associated with a fistula into the trachea
3. Stenosis

B. Inflammation
1. Reflux oesophagitis/peptic ulcer
2. Viral oesophagitis, e.g. influenza and herpes simplex
3. Fungal oesophagitis
   (i)   Moniliasis
   (ii) Aspergillosis
4. Uraemic oesophagitis
5. Corrosive chemical ingestion
6. Plummer-Vinson syndrome
7. Tuberculosis
8. Crohn's disease
9. Chagas' disease

C. Vascular disorders
Oesophageal varices

D. Mechanical disorders
1. Diverticula
   (i)   Traction
   (ii) Pulsion
2. Obstruction resulting from:
   (i)   Stricture—chronic peptic ulceration
   (ii)   Carcinoma
   (iii) Achalasia (cardiospasm)
   (iv)   Progressive systemic sclerosis
   (v)   Mucosal webs
   (vi)   Congenital stenosis
3. Rupture
   (i)   Mucosal (Mallory-Weiss syndrome)
   (ii) Full thickness—oesophageal perforation

4. Hiatus hernia
   (i) Sliding type
   (ii) Para-oesophageal (rolling) type

E. Benign tumours
1. Leiomyoma
2. Fibroma
3. Lipoma, etc

F. Malignant tumours
1. Carcinoma of the oesophagus
   Predisposing factors, many of which are speculative
   (i) Tobacco
   (ii) Alcohol
   (iii) Anatomical abnormalities, e.g. hiatus hernia, achalasia
   (iv) Lower socio-economic groups
   (v) Plummer-Vinson (postcricoid)
   (vi) Following corrosives
   Types
   (i) Squamous cell
   (ii) Adenocarcinoma, mainly at oesophago-gastric junction
       and arising from:
       Gastric epithelium at cardia,
       Columnar epithelium in lower 2 cm
       Submucosal glands
   (iii) Oat-cell
   Spread—Direct to:
   (i) Trachea or main bronchi
   (ii) Lung
   (iii) Mediastinum
   (iv) Aorta or heart (uncommon)
   Metastasis to:
   (i) Regional lymph nodes
   (ii) Liver
   (iii) Lungs
   (iv) Adrenals
   Prognosis
   5 year survival is below 10%
The remaining tumours are all very rare:
2. Sarcoma
   (i) Leiomyosarcoma
   (ii) Fibrosarcoma
3. Malignant melanoma
4. Carcino-sarcoma

STOMACH

A. Congenital
1. Diaphragmatic hernia
2. Congenital pyloric stenosis

B. Inflammations
1. Acute gastritis
   Causes
   (i) Alcohol excess
   (ii) Salicylates and other drugs
   (iii) Staphylococcal exotoxin in contaminated food
   (iv) Irritant chemicals/corrosives
   (v) After major surgery or trauma
2. Chronic gastritis
   (i) Superficial
      a. Degeneration and regeneration of the surface epithelium
      b. Inflammatory cell infiltration of the lamina propria
      c. Small intestinal metaplasia
   (ii) Atrophic
      a. Glandular atrophy
      b. Loss of specialised secretory cells
      c. Intestinal and pseudopyloric metaplasia
      d. Variable chronic inflammatory cell infiltration
3. Hypertrophic gastritis (Ménétrier's disease)
   (i) Rugal hypertrophy
   (ii) Cystic dilation of glands
   (iii) Strands of muscularis mucosae in lamina propria
   (iv) Variable hyperplasia of peptic and parietal cells
4. Eosinophilic gastritis
5. Crohn's 'gastritis'

C. Simple ulceration
1. Acute (stress) ulcers/erosions
   Predisposing factors
   (i) Aspirin
   (ii) Severe burns, major trauma, (Curling's ulcers)
   (iii) Cerebrovascular accidents, head injury
   (iv) Septicaemia
   (v) Uraemia
   (vi) ACTH or corticosteroid therapy
   (vii) Alcohol excess

2. Chronic peptic ulcers
    Sites
    (i)   Lesser curve and antrum
    (ii)   First part of duodenum
    (iii)   Lower oesophagus
    (iv)   Gastroenterostomy margins
    (v)   Meckel's diverticulum
    (vi)   Remainder of duodenum and jejunum in Zollinger-
            Ellison syndrome
    Predisposing factors
    (i)   Gastric ulceration
            a. Chronic gastritis
            b. Inherited factors (more frequent in blood group A)
            c. Increasing age
            d. Lower socio-economic class
    (ii)   Duodenal ulceration
            a. Hyperacidity and increased parietal cell mass
            b. Inheritance (increased in blood group O)
            c. Psychological factors
            d. Gastrin over-production (Z.E. syndrome)
            e. Increased incidence in patients with pulmonary
                emphysema
            f. Increased incidence in hyperparathyroidism
            g. Increased incidence in alcoholic cirrhosis
    Pathogenesis
    Chronic peptic ulcers occur when the digestive action of acid
    and pepsin overcome the natural defences of the mucosa
    (i)   Duodenal ulcers result in the great majority of cases
            from hyperacidity
    (ii)   Gastric ulcers are associated with normal or even low
            gastric acid levels and possibly result from bile reflux or
            lowered mucosal resistance due to:
            a. Diminished mucus secretion
            b. Mucosal ischaemia
            c. Slower epithelial renewal
    Complications
    (i)   Perforation
    (ii)   Haemorrhage
    (iii)   Stenosis
            a. Pyloric
            b. Hour-glass deformity
    (iv)   Malignant change

D. Benign tumours and polyps
1. Hyperplastic (regenerative) polyps
2. True neoplasms
   - (i) Adenoma
   - (ii) Leiomyoma
   - (iii) Lipoma
   - (iv) Haemangioma
   - (v) Neurilemmoma/Neurofibroma
3. Hamartomas and heterotopias
   - (i) Heterotopic pancreas
   - (ii) Adenomyoma (myo-epithelial hamartoma)
   - (iii) Peutz-Jegher's polyps
   - (iv) Cronkhite-Canada syndrome
     - a. Polyposis of the stomach and intestines
     - b. Abnormal skin pigmentation
     - c. Nail dystrohy
     - d. Baldness

E. Malignant tumours
1. Carcinoma
   Precancerous conditions
     - a. Pernicious anaemia/atrophic gastritis
     - b. Adenomatous polyps
   (Chronic peptic ulcer →less than 1% gastric carcinomas)
   Types
   - (i) Nodular
   - (ii) Ulcerative
   - (iii) Polypoid or fungating
   - (iv) Linitis plastica
   - (v) Superficial carcinoma
   Microscopic appearances
   - (i) Intra-mucosal (carcinoma-in-situ)
   - (ii) Adenocarcinoma
   - (iii) Anaplastic carcinoma
   Spread
   - (i) Direct to pancreas, liver, colon etc
   - (ii) Lymphatic to nodes along lesser and then greater curve
   - (iii) Blood spread to liver, lung, skin
   - (iv) Transcoelomic to omentum, peritoneum and ovaries (Krukenberg spread)
2. Carcinoid tumour
3. Lymphoma
4. Leiomyosarcoma
5. Fibrosarcoma
6. Adeno-acanthoma

SMALL INTESTINE
A. Congenital
1. Duodenal diverticula
2. Diverticulosis of jejunum and ileum
3. Meckel's diverticulum
4. Atresia
5. Failures of rotation

B. Inflammation/ulceration
1. Crohn's disease (regional enteritis)
   Sites—most cases seen in the small intestine but can involve any part from mouth to anus
   Gross features
   (i) 'Hosepipe' thickening of wall
   (ii) Ulcers—aphthoid or linear
   (iii) Deep fissures
   (iv) 'Cobblestone' mucosa
   (v) Skip lesions
   (vi) Enlarged lymph nodes
   Microscopic appearances
   (i) Granulomata (sarcoid-type)
   (ii) Transmural inflammation
   (iii) Aggregated pattern of inflammatory cells
   (iv) Submucosal oedema, lymphangiectasia, and fibrosis
   (v) Fissures
   (vi) Neuromatoid hyperplasia
   Complications
   (i) Malabsorption
   (ii) Obstruction
   (iii) Fistula formation
   (iv) Perforation
   (v) Haemorrhage
   (vi) Liver disease—peribiliary fibrosis
   (vii) Skin lesions
   (viii) Ocular inflammation
   (ix) Malignancy (?)
2. Infective causes
   (i) Cholera
   (ii) E. coli infections in infants
   (iii) Typhoid/paratyphoid
   (iv) Staphylococcal enterocolitis
   (v) Tuberculosis
   (vi) Actinomycosis
   (vii) Viral diseases
      a. Enteroviruses
      b. Adenoviruses
   (viii) ? Whipple's disease

(ix)   Giardiasis—found more commonly in:
Childhood
Malnutrition
Following gastrectomy
Pancreatic disease
Hypogammaglobulinaemia
Nodular lymphoid hyperplasia
Dysgammaglobulinaemia

C. Malabsorption

Due to abnormal small intestinal function:
1.   Villous atrophy
Terminology
(i)   Villous architecture
a. Mild, moderate or severe partial villous atrophy
b. Total villous atrophy
(ii)   Crypt cellularity and mitotic activity
a. Crypt hyperplasia
b. Crypt hypoplasia
Causes of Crypt hyperplastic villous atrophy
(i)   Coeliac disease:
caused by an abnormal response of the small intestinal
mucosa to an unknown peptide found in the wheat
protein, gluten. This is likely to be immunologically
mediated.
Immunological findings
a. Mucosal plasma cells show diminished IgA, and
increased IgM secretion
b. IgM is decreased in the serum whilst IgA is increased
c. Features of immune dysfunction such as splenic
atrophy and impaired lymphocyte transformation
d. The serum may contain IgM antibodies to certain
fractions of gluten
e. IgA deposited on basement-membrane following
gluten challenge. IgG deposits found in untreated
coeliacs
Microscopic features
a. Total or severe partial villous atrophy
b. Cuboidal surface epithelium with palisading of nuclei
and indistinct brush border
c. Heavy infiltration of epithelium by theliolymphocytes
d. Increase in lymphocytes and plasma cells in lamina
propria

Complications
   a. Lymphoma
   b. Ulcerative jejunitis
  (ii) Tropical sprue
  (iii) Dermatitis herpetiformis
  (iv) Postinfective malabsorption syndrome
  (v) Carcinomatosis
  (vi) Diabetes mellitus
  (vii) Neomycin (?)
Causes of Crypt hypoplastic villous atrophy
  (i) Pernicious anaemia
  (ii) Folic acid deficiency
  (iii) Carcinomatosis
  (iv) Hypopituitarism
  (v) Irradiation
  (vi) Paneth-cell deficiency (?)

2. Biochemical disorders
  (i) Sucrase—isomaltase deficiency
  (ii) Lactase deficiency
  (iii) Monosaccharide malabsorption
  (iv) Hartnup disease
  (v) Cystinuria
  (vi) Congenital chlorodiarrhoea
  (vii) Abeta-lipoproteinaemia

3. Lymphatic abnormalities
  (i) Intestinal lymphangiectasia
  (ii) Whipple's disease

4. Disease of the intestinal wall
  (i) Amyloidosis
  (ii) Radiation injury
  (iii) Collagen diseases
  (iv) Crohn's disease

5. Altered bacterial flora
  (i) Stagnant loop syndrome
  (ii) Jejunal diverticulosis
  (iii) Multiple strictures ⎫
  (iv) Fistulae ⎭ as in Crohn's disease

6. Vascular—
  small intestinal ischaemia

D. Vascular disorders
1. Mucosal vessels
   - (i) Acute haemorrhagic gastroenteritis
   - (ii) Hereditary haemorrhagic telangectasia
2. Mesenteric arteries
   - (i) Thrombosis/embolus
   - (ii) Atherosclerosis alone
   - (iii) Fibro-muscular hyperplasia
   - (iv) Polyarteritis nodosa
3. Mesenteric veins
   - (i) Thrombosis
   - (ii) Strangulation (in later stages leads to arterial occlusion)

Arterial and venous occlusion results in haemorrhagic infarction.

4. Non-occlusive ischaemia resulting from
   - (i) Cardiac failure
   - (ii) Shock
   - (iii) Drug-induced vasoconstriction

E. Mechanical disorders
Obstruction of the small intestine

Causes
- (i) Hernias
- (ii) Adhesions
- (iii) Neoplasms
- (iv) Intussusception
- (v) Volvulus
- (vi) Strictures, congenital or acquired
- (vii) Atresia
- (viii) Gall stones or foreign bodies (including food bolus)
- (ix) Meconium plug (mucoviscidosis)

Obstruction may also result from mesenteric thrombosis and neurogenic paralytic ileus.

F. Benign tumours
1. Adenoma/papilloma
2. Leiomyoma (difficult to exclude malignancy, better termed 'smooth muscle tumour')
3. Fibroma
4. Lipoma
5. Haemangioma (may be part of the Osler-Rendu-Weber syndrome)
6. Lymphangioma
7. Peutz-Jegher's polyps

G. Malignant tumours
1. Adenocarcinoma (uncommon)
2. Carcinoid tumour
3. Lymphoma
4. Leiomyosarcoma

APPENDIX

A. Inflammation
1. Acute non-specific
   Predisposing factors (act mainly by causing obstruction)
   (i) Lymphoid hyperplasia
      a. Physiological
      b. Measles and other viral diseases
   (ii) Faecolith/Foreign bodies/Food residues
   (iii) Mucosal oedema
   (iv) Diverticulosis of the appendix
   (v) Carcinoid tumour
   (vi) Threadworms
   Complications
   (i) Perforation leading to:
      a. Generalised peritonitis
      b. Appendicular abscess
      c. Fistula formation
   (ii) Suppurative pylephlebitis and liver abscess
   (iii) Septicaemia
   (iv) Chronic appendicitis
   (v) Mucocoele which may rupture and produce myxoma peritonei
2. Yersinia enterocolitica appendicitis
3. Typhoid
4. Tuberculosis
5. Crohn's disease
6. Actinomycosis
7. Starch-grain granulomatosis
8. Polyarteritis nodosa
9. Eosinophil granuloma

B. Neoplasms
1. Carcinoid tumour
2. Adenocarcinoma
3. Lymphoma

LARGE INTESTINE

A. Congenital
1. Atresia including imperforate anus
2. Stenosis
3. Duplication
4. Hirschsprung's disease—aganglionosis

B. Inflammation
1. Infective agents
   (i) Bacillary dysentery (Shigellosis)
   (ii) Typhoid/paratyphoid
   (iii) Tuberculosis
   (iv) Staphylococcal enterocolitis
   (v) Amoebic dysentery
   (vi) Schistosomiasis
   (vii) Balantidiasis
   (viii) Actinomycosis
   (ix) Rectal venereal diseases
      a. Gonorrhoea
      b. Syphilis
      c. Lymphogranuloma venereum
2. Ulcerative colitis
   Sites
   Usually starts in rectum and spreads proximally to involve the entire colon
   Gross features
   (i) Continuity of involvement
   (ii) Confluent irregular ulcers
   (iii) 'Pseudopolyps'—residual inflamed mucosa
   (iv) Intense vascularity
   Microscopic features
   (i) Continuous inflammation maximal in the mucosa
   (ii) Congestion and vasodilatation
   (iii) Crypt abscesses
   (iv) Undermining ulcers and inflammatory polyps
   (v) Glandular atrophy and irregularity in healed areas
   (vi) Mucin depletion
   (vii) Paneth-cell metaplasia
   (viii) Pre-malignant dysplasia may be present
   Complications
   (i) Haemorrhage
   (ii) Anaemia
   (iii) Electrolyte disturbances
   (iv) Perforation
   (v) Toxic dilatation
   (vi) Malignant change—carcinoma
   (vii) Extra-intestinal disease
      a. Skin lesions—pyoderma gangrenosum, erythema nodosum
      b. Arthritis/ankylosing spondylitis
      c. Liver disease—chronic pericholangitis
      d. Eye disease—iritis, uveitis, episcleritis
      e. Amyloidosis
3. Crohn's colitis
4. Irradiation colitis
5. Pseudomembranous colitis
6. Uraemic enterocolitis

E. Vascular disorder

1. Ischaemia
   The causes of ischaemia are the same as those in the small intestine.
   Ischaemia results in:
   (i)   Infarction
   (ii) Ischaemic colitis
       a. Membranous colitis
       b. Stricture
2. Haemorrhoids
   Varicosities of the superior and inferior rectal veins.
   Causes
   (i)   Chronic constipation
   (ii) Heavy physical work
   (iii) Pregnancy
   (iv) Pelvic tumours
   (v)   Portal hypertension
   (vi) Rectal carcinoma

F. Mechanical disorders

1. Diverticular disease
2. Volvulus
3. Herniation
4. Intussusception

G. Benign tumours and polyps

1. Epithelial
   (i)   Tubular adenoma (adenomatous polyp)
   (ii) Villo-tubular adenoma
   (iii) Villous adenoma
   (iv) Metaplastic polyps
2. Lymphoid
   (i)   Benign lymphoid polyp
3. Connective tissues
   (i)   Lipoma
   (ii) Smooth muscle tumours
   (iii) Neurogenic
4. Mixed (harmartoma)
   (i)   Peutz-Jegher's polyps
   (ii) Juvenile polyposis

H. Malignant Tumours
1. Carcinoma
   Aetiology
   (i) Genetic—some familial tendency
   (ii) Chronic inflammation—ulcerative colitis
   (iii) Dietary factors
      a. ? Bile salts and anaerobic organisms
      b. ? Low residue food
   (iv) Polyps
   Gross features
   (i) Annular ulcer
   (ii) Polypoid/fungating
   Microscopic appearances
   (i) Adenocarcinoma—glandular
   (ii) Mucoid (colloid) carcinoma
   (iii) Undifferentiated carcinoma
      and in the lower rectum and anal canal
   (iv) Squamous carcinoma (including basaloid variety)
   (v) Basal cell carcinoma
   (vi) Muco-epidermoid carcinoma
   Spread—
   Dukes' classification—
      Stage A—confined to the wall of the colon/rectum
      Stage B—extends into surrounding fat but there is no
      involvement of regional lymph glands
      Stage C—secondary deposits present in the regional
      glands
      Stage D—distant metastases
   Blood spread is mainly to liver and lungs
   Complications
   (i) Obstruction
   (ii) Perforation
   (iii) Fistula formation
   (iv) Haemorrhoids (rectal)
   (v) Anaemia
   (vi) Diarrhoea
2. Carcinoid tumour
3. Lymphoma
4. Sarcoma
   (i) leiomyosarcoma
   (ii) fibrosarcoma
5. Malignant melanoma (anal region)

FURTHER READING

Creamer, B. (Ed.) (1974) *The Small Intestine.* Tutorials in
Postgraduate Medicine, 4. London: Heinemann.

Ming, Si Chun (1973) Tumors of the Eosophagus and Stomach.
Atlas of Tumor Pathology, 2nd series, 11. Montvale, N.J.:
A.F.I.P.S. Press.

Mottet, K.N. (1971) Histopathological spectrum of regional enteritis
and ulcerative colitis. *Major Problems in Pathology,* **2.**
Philadelphia: W.B. Saunders.

Morson, B.C. & Dawson, I.M.P. (1972) *Gastro-Intestinal Pathology.*
Oxford: Blackwell.

Thackray, A.C. & Lucas, R.B. (1974) Tumors of the Major Salivary
Glands. *Atlas of Tumor Pathology,* 2nd series, 10. Montvale,
N.J.: A.F.I.P.S. Press.

Whitehead, R. (1973) *Mucosal Biopsy of the Gastro-Intestinal Tract.*
Philadelphia: W.B. Saunders.

Liver, gall-bladder and pancreas

DISEASES OF THE LIVER

A. Congenital
1. Accessory lobes—Riedel's lobe
2. Congenital cystic disease (found in association with polycystic kidneys)
3. Congenital hepatic fibrosis

B. Inflammations
1. Viral hepatitis

   Types
   (i) Hepatitis A caused by an RNA virus—short incubation, epidemic
   (ii) Hepatitis B
       Dane particle—complete virion consisting of a core containing circular DNA formed in liver cell nuclei and a double shelled coat which is formed in the cytoplasm and is often found detached from the core. The core antigen is termed HB_cAg and the surface antigen, HB_sAg. A third antigen—*antigen e,* is associated with hepatitis-B-specific DNA polymerase.
   (iii) Miscellaneous viral diseases involving the liver include
       a. Infectious mononucleosis
       b. Cytomegalovirus
       c. Herpes hominis
       d. Yellow fever

   Microscopic features of hepatitis A and B are indistinguishable
   (i) Necrosis of hepatocytes, usually single-cell but may be zonal
   (ii) Other degenerative changes—'ballooning'
   (iii) Inflammatory cell infiltration of portal tracts and parenchyma, mainly lymphocytes with small numbers of polymorphs
   (iv) Kupffer cell proliferation
   (v) Variable cholestasis
   (vi) Features of regeneration

Variants of acute viral hepatitis
   (i)   Anicteric hepatitis
   (ii) Cholestatic hepatitis
   (iii) Subacute hepatic necrosis with bridging between
         adjacent central veins and portal tracts
   (iv) Massive hepatic necrosis
Fate of acute viral hepatitis
   (i)   Resolution
   (ii) Recurrence of acute hepatitis
   (iii) Chronic persistent hepatitis
   (iv) Chronic agressive hepatitis (chronic active)
   (v)   Cirrhosis
2. Bacterial infection
   (i)   Tuberculosis especially in miliary spread
   (ii) Brucellosis
3. Spirochaetes
   (i)   Syphilis
         a. Congenital pericellular fibrosis
         b. Gummata—hepar lobatum
   (ii) Borrelia recurrentis infection
   (iii) Leptospirosis (Weil's disease)
4. Protozoa
   (i)   Amoebiasis
         a. Amoebic hepatitis
         b. Amoebic abscess
   (ii) Toxoplasmosis
5. Rickettsia
   (i)   Q fever
6. Fungi
   (i)   Histoplasmosis
7. Parasites
   (i)   Hydatid cysts
   (ii) Clonorchis sinensis
8. Non-specific inflammation
   (i)   Abscess (pyaemic)
   (ii) Cholangitis

C. Drugs and the liver

Drugs may injure the liver by a direct toxic effect or because of an
idiosyncratic reaction where the drug is acting as an allergen. Four
major categories of liver damage are produced:
   1. Direct hepatic necrosis
   2. Hepatitis-like reactions
   3. Cholestasis and hepatitis
   4. Cholestasis alone

1. *Direct hepatic necrosis.* This is usually a predictable injury resulting in zonal or massive necrosis.
> *Causes include*
> (i) Paracetamol (acetaminophen) in acute overdosage
> (ii) Ferrous sulphate in acute overdosage
> (iii) Carbon tetrachloride and benzene derivatives
> (iv) Methotrexate and 6-mercaptopurine (non-zonal)
> (v) Aflatoxin
> (vi) Tannic acid

2. *Hepatitis-like reactions.* These are hypersensitivity reactions and may produce a histological picture indistinguishable from acute viral hepatitis or a chronic aggressive hepatitis.
> *Causes include*
> (i) Halothane
> (ii) Monoamine oxidase inhibitors
> (iii) α-Methyldopa
> (iv) Isoniazid
> (v) Oxyphenisatin

3. *Cholestasis and hepatitis.* This also represents a hypersensitivity reaction in which cholestasis is the major feature but some histological evidence of hepatitis is usually present.
> *Causes include*
> (i) Phenothiazines especially Chlorpromazine
> (ii) Tricyclic antidepressants
> (iii) Anxiolytic drugs (Chlordiazepoxide, Diazepam)
> (iv) Anti-inflammatory drugs (Phenylbutazone, Indomethacin)
> (v) Anti-tuberculous drugs (PAS, rifampicin)
> (vi) Antibiotics (Erythromycin, Sulphamethoxazole)

4. *Cholestasis alone.* This injury is not related to hypersensitivity but genetic factors may alter susceptibility:
> *Causes*
> (i) Anabolic steroids (methyltestosterone/norethandrolone)
> (ii) Contraceptive steroids

5. Miscellaneous drug injuries
> (i) Diffuse fatty liver—tetracycline
> (ii) Increase in liver cell lipofuscins—phenacetin
> (iii) Fatty change, fibrosis, and cirrhosis—long-term methotrexate therapy for psoriasis
> (iv) Central vein occlusion—Senecio alkaloids, urethane
> (v) Peliosis hepatitis (haemorrhagic cysts)—anabolic steroids
> (vi) Granulomata—phenylbutazone

6. Alcohol and the liver
    (i)   Fatty liver—may be associated with:
        a. Jaundice
        b. Portal hypertension
        c. Encephalopathy
        d. Fat embolism (very rare)
    (ii) Alcoholic hepatitis
    Features
        a. Centrilobular single-cell necrosis
        b. Mallory's hyaline bodies
        c. Fatty change
        d. Polymorph infiltration
        e. Pericellular collagenisation
        with or without cirrhosis
    (iii) Cirrhosis
    (iv) Portal fibrosis
    (v) Chronic aggressive hepatitis

D. **Degenerative/metabolic disorders**
  1. Brown atrophy—lipofuscinosis
  2. Fatty change
    (i)   Diabetes mellitus
    (ii) Starvation
    (iii) Alcoholic
    (iv) Obesity
    (v) Kwashiorkor
    (vi) Drugs—methotrexate, corticosteroids
    (vii) Reye's syndrome (? viral aetiology)
        a. Fever/vomiting
        b. Hypoglycaemia
        c. Respiratory acidosis
        d. Encephalopathy
  3. Amyloidosis—usually secondary type
  4. Glycogen deposition
    (i)   Diabetes mellitus (with nuclear vacuolation)
    (ii) von Gierke's disease
  5. Lipid storage
    (i)   Hand-Schüller-Christian disease
    (ii) Gaucher's disease
    (iii) Niemann-Pick
  6. Haemosiderosis/Haemochromatosis
  7. Wilson's disease

E. Vascular disorders
1. Portal hypertension follows obstruction to the portal blood flow somewhere along its course
   (i) Extrahepatic portal vein
      a. Thrombosis possibly secondary to pancreatitis or pylephlebitis
      b. Pressure from glands in porta hepatis
      c. Invasion by carcinoma of pancreas or biliary tract
      d. Stricture or ligature following surgery
   (ii) Intrahepatic portal veins
      a. Schistosomiasis
      b. Infiltration of portal tracts by lymphoma, myeloproliferative disease, or sarcoidosis
      c. Congenital hepatic fibrosis
      d. Obliterative portal venopathy
   (iii) Sinusoids or small hepatic veins
      a. Cirrhosis
      b. Veno-occlusive disease resulting from ingestion of Senecio alkaloids, administration of cytotoxic drugs and liver irradiation
   (iv) Hepatic veins (Budd-Chiari syndrome)
      a. Thrombosis
      b. Tumour involvement
   (v) Chronic venous congestion of liver (CVC)
      a. Congestive cardiac failure
      b. Constrictive pericarditis
      c. Tricuspid incompetance
2. Infarcts resulting from occlusion of the hepatic arteries are uncommon and usually result from a severe arteritis or when the additional supply from the portal vein is diminished. Occlusion of intrahepatic branches of the portal vein results in haemorrhagic lesions—'Zahn's infarcts'.
3. Hypoxic centrilobular necrosis is seen in shock.
4. Cardiac 'cirrhosis'
   Prolonged and severe CVC leads to centrilobular necrosis, distortion of reticulin framework and scarring. In the most severe cases this scarring may link-up adjacent central veins to produce 'reverse lobulation'. The intervening parenchyma rarely shows sufficient evidence of regeneration to justify the term cirrhosis.

F. Cirrhosis
A combination of widespread fibrosis and regenerative nodule formation following necrosis of liver cells.
   Aetiological classification
   1. Cryptogenic
   2. Alcoholic
   3. Viral hepatitis (including neonatal hepatitis)
   4. Immunologically mediated
      (i) Chronic active hepatitis
      (ii) Primary biliary cirrhosis

5. Infiltrations associated with fibrosis
    (i) Haemochromatosis
    (ii) Wilson's disease
    (iii) Schistosomiasis (pipe-stem cirrhosis)
6. Biliary obstruction
    Secondary biliary cirrhosis
7. Chronic venous congestion
    Cardiac 'cirrhosis'
8. Metabolic and inherited disorders
    (i) α-1-antitrypsin deficiency
    (ii) Mucoviscidosis
    (iii) Hereditary haemorrhagic telangiectasia
    (iv) Galactosaemia
    (v) Hereditary fructose intolerance
9. Drug-induced or toxins
    (i) Methotrexate
    (ii) Aflatoxin

Complications of cirrhosis
1. Hepatocellular failure
    (i) Increasing jaundice
    (ii) Coagulopathy
    (iii) Encephalopathy
2. Portal hypertension
    (i) Splenomegaly
    (ii) Enlargement of porto-systemic anastomoses
    (iii) Ascites
3. Development of liver-cell carcinoma
4. Intercurrent infection e.g. suppurative peritonitis

G. Benign tumours
1. Cavernous haemangioma (hamartoma)
2. Adenoma
    (i) Bile duct adenoma
    (ii) Liver cell adenoma (associated with contraceptive steroids)
3. Mesenchymal hamartoma
4. Infantile haemangioendothelioma

H. Malignant tumours
1. Liver cell carcinoma
    Predisposing factors
    (i) Cirrhosis, especially haemochromatosis
    (ii) Aflatoxins?
    (iii) Hepatitis B antigen?
2. Bile duct carcinoma
    Predisposing factors
    (i) Thorotrast
    (ii) Clonorchis sinensis infestation
    (iii) Arsenic
4. Hepatoblastoma
5. Lymphoma
6. Fibrosarcoma/neurogenic sarcoma (very rare)

DISEASES OF THE GALL-BLADDER
A. Congenital
1. Atresia of the gall-bladder or of any part of the hepatic or common bile ducts
2. Folded gall bladder
3. Complete or incomplete septum across the lumen
4. 'Floating' gall-bladder
5. Anomalies of the cystic duct and artery
6. Choledocal cyst

B. Inflammation
1. Acute cholecystitis
   Results
   (i) Resolution
   (ii) Empyema
   (iii) Gangrene which may perforate and produce
       a. Generalised peritonitis
       b. Local abscess
   (iv) Ascending cholangitis
2. Chronic cholecystitis
   Features
   (i) Fibrosis
   (ii) Mucosal herniations (Aschoff-Rokitansky sinuses)
   (iii) Chronic inflammatory cell infiltrate
   (iv) Muscular hypertrophy

C. Cholelithiasis
Factors involved
(i) Production of an abnormal bile
    a. Excess bile pigment
    b. Excess of cholesterol relative to bile salts and lecithin
(ii) Infection and inflammation
(iii) Stasis
Composition
(i) Mixed stones (about 90%)
(ii) Pure stones
    a. Cholesterol
    b. Calcium bilirubinate
    c. Calcium carbonate
Effects
(i) Clinically 'silent'
(ii) Inflammation—provoke acute and chronic cholecystitis
(iii) Obstruction
    a. Cystic duct; leading to empyema and mucocoele
    b. Common bile duct; producing obstructive jaundice
    c. Ampulla of Vater; jaundice and in some cases acute pancreatitis
(iv) Erosion and perforation
    a. Biliary peritonitis
    b. Gall-stone ileus
(v) Malignant change
    Gall-stones are present in about 90% of cases of carcinoma of the gall-bladder

D. Mechanical disorders
1. Diverticulosis of the gall-bladder
    - (i) Fundal, usually in relation to a congenital septum (so-called 'adenomyoma')
    - (ii) Generalised—'cholecystitis glandularis proliferans'
2. Obstruction to the extra-hepatic bile ducts
    - (i) Gall-stones
    - (ii) Benign stricture
        - a. Following surgery
        - b. Traumatic
        - c. Fibrosis around a peptic ulcer
        - d. Chronic pancreatitis
        - e. Benign bile duct tumours
        - f. Sclerosing cholangitis
    - (iii) External pressure
        - a. Carcinoma of the pancreas
        - b. Enlarged lymph glands at the porta hepatis
        - c. Duodenal diverticulum
    - (iv) Malignant stricture/occlusion
        - a. Carcinoma of the Ampulla
        - b. Carcinoma of the bile ducts
        - c. Invasion by neighbouring carcinoma
    - (v) Atresia

E. Benign tumours
1. Papilloma
2. Adenoma
3. Papillary adenomatosis (widespread)

F. Malignant tumours
Carcinoma
- (i) Gall-bladder
    Gross features
    - a. Papillary
    - b. Diffuse infiltration
    Microscopic appearances
    - a. Adenocarcinoma
    - b. Squamous carcinoma (metaplasia)
    - c. Anaplastic
- (ii) Extrahepatic ducts
    Gross features
    - a. Papillary nodule
    - b. Thickening of the wall
    Microscopical appearances
    - a. Papillary adenocarcinoma
    - b. Scirrhous, mucous-secreting adenocarcinoma

DISEASES OF THE PANCREAS

A. Congenital

1. Ectopic pancreas in
   - (i) Stomach and duodenum
   - (ii) Jejunum
   - (iii) Meckel's diverticulum
   - (iv) Ileum
2. Anomalies of the ducts
3. Annular pancreas
4. Mucoviscidosis (cystic fibrosis)
   Lesions mainly due to exocrine gland obstruction by secretions.
   Pathogenesis unknown
   Autosomal recessive inheritance
   Lesions
   - (i) Meconium ileus
   - (ii) Pancreas—fibrocystic changes
   - (iii) Lungs—recurrent bronchopneumonia usually Staphylococcal
   - (iv) Liver—biliary cirrhosis
   - (v) Salivary glands—acinar atrophy and fibrosis

B. Inflammations

1. Acute haemorrhagic pancreatitis
   Aetiological factors
   - (i) Alcohol excess
   - (ii) Bile reflux—biliary tract disease and gall-stones
   - (iii) Hypersecretion and obstruction
   - (iv) Duodenal reflux
   A small proportion of cases are associated with:
   - (i) Hypothermia in the aged
   - (ii) Mumps
   - (iii) Primary hyperparathyroidism
   - (iv) Hyperlipoproteinaemia
   - (v) Pregnancy and gall-stones
   - (vi) Trauma
   - (vii) Carcinoma of the pancreas
   - (viii) Corticosteroid and azathioprine therapy
   Effects (in severe cases)
   - (i) Hypovolaemic shock
   - (ii) Paralytic ileus
   - (iii) Hypocalcaemia
   - (iv) Hypomagnesaemia
   - (v) Tetany
   Results
   - (i) Resolution, usually incomplete
   - (ii) Abscess
   - (iii) Pseudocyst formation in lesser-sac
   - (iv) Recurrent acute pancreatitis
   - (v) Chronic pancreatitis

2. Chronic pancreatitis
   Aetiology
   (i)   Idiopathic
   (ii)   Alcohol excess
   (iii) Following acute pancreatitis
   (iv)   Primary hyperparathyroidism
   (v)   Biliary tract disease
   (vi)   Haemochromatosis
   Effects
   (i)   Exocrine insufficiency— steatorrhoea
   (ii)   Diabetes mellitus
   (iii) Obstructive jaundice
   (iv)   Haematemesis and melaena

C. Degenerative disorders
1. Fatty infiltration (adiposity)
2. Atrophy
   (i)   Atherosclerotic
   (ii)   Obstruction of major ducts resulting from
          a. Atresia or congenital stenosis
          b. Pancreatic calculi
          c. Squamous metaplasia
          d. Carcinoma involving ducts
          e. Ligature
          f. Inflammatory stenosis
3. Acinar ectasia in uraemia

D. Benign Tumours
1. Adenoma and cystadenoma
2. Fibroma
3. Lipoma
4. Haemangioma

E. Carcinoma of the pancreas
Microscopic types
1. Adenocarcinoma
   (i)   Mucous-secreting (duct origin)
   (ii)   Acinar, non-mucous secreting
2. Anaplastic (uncommon)
Complications
1. Biliary obstruction
   (i)   Obstructive jaundice
   (ii)   Cholangitis
   (iii) Biliary cirrhosis
2. Invasion of duodenum—bleeding
3. Diabetes mellitus
4. Venous thrombosis
   (i)   Portal vein
   (ii)   Thrombophlebitis migrans
5. Chronic pancreatitis

6. Excessive lipase secretion by widespread tumour may give
   (i)   Polyarthritis
   (ii) Panniculitis (fat necrosis)
   (iii) Eosinophilia
7. Myopathy/peripheral neuropathy
8. Thrombotic endocarditis
9. Fibrinolysis and haemorrhage

F. Islet cell tumours
   1. Insulinoma (ß-cell tumour)
      Usually solitary but in about 10% of cases are multiple. 10 –
      15% are malignant
   2. Gastrinoma (delta-cell tumour) associated with the Zollinger-
      Ellison syndrome
      About 60% are malignant

FURTHER READING

Scheuer, P.J. (1973) *Liver Biopsy Interpretation,* 2nd edn. London:
    Baillière Tindall.
Sherlock, S. (1975) *Diseases of the Liver and Biliary System,* 5th
    edn. Oxford: Blackwell.
Walker, R. & Mallinson, C. (1972) Disorders of the pancreas.
    Medicine, **8,** 598.
Weinbren, K. (1975) Diseases of the liver. In *Recent Advances in
    Pathology* 9, eds. Harrison, C.V. & Weinbren, K. p. 97.
    Edinburgh: Churchill Livingstone.

Cardiovascular system

PERICARDIUM

A. Inflammation
1. Acute pericarditis
   (i) Secondary to myocardial infarction
   (ii) Uraemia
   (iii) Rheumatic fever
   (iv) Infectious causes
      a. Bacterial—staphylococcal, pneumococcal
      b. Viral—especially Coxsackie B.
      c. Tuberculous
      d. Fungal
   (v) Drug reactions
   (vi) Postmyocardial infarction/Postcardiotomy syndromes
   (vii) Idiopathic
2. Chronic pericarditis
   (i) Tuberculous
   (ii) Rheumatoid disease
   (iii) SLE
   (iv) Systemic sclerosis
   (v) Idiopathic constrictive pericarditis
   (vi) Actinomycosis
   (vii) Amoebiasis

B. Tumours of the pericardium
1. Secondary carcinoma, spread from:
   (i) Bronchus
   (ii) Oesophagus
   (iii) Breast
2. Lymphoma/leukaemia may involve pericardium
3. Invasion by thymoma
4. Mesothelioma

HEART

A. Congenital

1. Disorders of the entire heart
   - (i) Dextrocardia—with or without situs inversus
   - (ii) Laevocardia
   - (iii) Cardiomegaly
     Causes
     - a. Shunts
     - b. Anomalies of the coronary arteries
     - c. Myocarditis
     - d. Obstructive cardiomyopathy
     - e. Infantile endocardial fibroelastosis
     - f. Hereditary diseases—Friedreich's ataxia, Refsum's syndrome
     - g. Storage disorders—Glycogen storage (Pompe's disease)
   - (iv) Congenital 'rhabdomyomas', as in tuberous sclerosis
2. Acyanotic shunts (left-right)
   - (i) Ventricular septal defect (VSD)
   - (ii) Atrial septal defect (ASD)
   - (iii) Patent ductus arteriosus
3. Cyanotic shunts (right-left)
   - (i) Tetralogy of Fallot
     - a. Pulmonary stenosis
     - b. Ventricular septal defect
     - c. Dextraposition and over-riding of the aorta
     - d. Right ventricular hypertrophy
   - (ii) Eisenmenger complex
     VSD with reversal of shunt resulting from pulmonary hypertension
   - (iii) Transposition of the great vessels
4. Valvular abnormalities
   - (i) Pulmonary stenosis
   - (ii) Pulmonary atresia (+ VSD)
   - (iii) Bicuspid aortic valve
   - (iv) Aortic stenosis
   - (v) Atresia of the aorta
   - (vi) Tricuspid atresia (+ ASD)
   - (vii) Ebstein's anomaly—malformation of the tricuspid with downward displacement of the valve
   - (viii) Bicuspid 'tricuspid' valve
   - (ix) Mitral atresia (+ ASD)
   - (x) 'Ballooning' of mitral valve cusps
   - (xi) 'Floppy-valve syndrome' sometimes associated with Marfan's syndrome
5. Coarctation of the aorta

B. Myocarditis
Cardiomyopathy of inflammatory nature caused by
1. Rheumatic fever
2. Viral diseases
    (i)   Coxsackie B
    (ii)   Echo virus
    (iii) Poliomyelitis
    (iv)   Mumps
    (v)   Measles
    (vi)   Infectious mononucleosis
    (vii) Psittacosis
    (vii) Variola
3. Bacterial infections
    (i)   Diphtheria
    (ii)   Typhoid
    (iii) Spread from infective endocarditis
    (iv)   Pyaemic spread, staph. streptococci, etc.
4. Parasitic diseases
    (i)   Toxoplasmosis
    (ii)   Trichinosis
    (iii) Trypanosomiasis (Chagas' disease)
5. Acute iodipathic myocarditis (Fiedler's)
    (i)   Diffuse interstitial form
    (ii)   Giant-cell (tuberculoid) form
6. Sarcoidosis
7. Syphilis

C. Cardiomyopathy
Myocardial disorders of obscure aetiology.
1. Congestive cardiomyopathy
    Aetiology
    (i)   Idiopathic
    (ii)   Familial
    (iii) Alcoholic (cobalt in beer ?)
    (iv)   Associated with skeletal myopathies, e.g. Duchenne-
           type, Friedreich's ataxia
    (v)   Post-partum
2. Hypertrophic obstructive cardiomyopathy
    (i)   Familial—transmitted as an autosomal dominant
    (ii)   Sporadic (idiopathic)
    Forms
    (i)   Superior thickening of the septum causing left
           ventricular outflow obstruction
    (ii)   Diffuse involvement of left and right ventricles and lower
           part of the septum causing resistance to ventricular
           filling—inflow obstruction
3. Obliterative cardiomyopathy (endomyocardial fibrosis)
    Results in
    (i)   Mitral incompetence
    (ii)   Atrial dilatation and ball thrombi
    (iii) Pulmonary hypertension

D. Myocardial involvement in generalised disorders
(Sometimes referred to as secondary cardiomyopathy)
1.   Storage diseases
     (i)   Glycogen storage (Pompe's)
     (ii)   Refsum's disease
     (iii)   Niemann-Pick's disease
2.   Amyloidosis
3.   Collagen diseases
     (i)   Rheumatoid disease
     (ii)   Progressive systemic sclerosis
     (iii)   SLE
     (iv)   Polyarteritis nodosa
4.   Haemochromatosis
5.   Beri-beri heart disease
6.   Chemicals and drugs, e.g. emetine, chloroform, glycosides
7.   Potassium and magnesium depletion
8.   Endocrine disorders
     (i)   Acromegaly
     (ii)   Myxoedema

E.   Rheumatic fever
Aetiology. An allergic reaction to streptococcal antigens
1.   ? Antibodies to these antigens cross-react with myocardial
     fibres, arterial smooth-muscle cells, and connective tissue
     glycoproteins
2.   ?? Immune complexes are formed which are deposited at the
     site of the lesions.
The Aschoff nodule
1.   Fibrinoid degeneration of collagen
2.   Mixed inflammatory cells
3.   Large mesenchymal cells (Anitschkow myocytes) which are
     probably altered fibroblasts
4.   Occasional Aschoff giant-cells
Lesions
1.   Heart
     (i)   Pericarditis—'bread and butter' type
     (ii)   Myocarditis
     (iii)   Endocarditis
             Valvulitis with vegetations
             a. Mitral
             b. Aortic
             c. Pulmonary (uncommon)
     (iv)   Chronic deformity
             a. Mitral stenosis/incompetence
             b. Aortic stenosis/incompetence
     (v)   Atrial fibrillation
2.   Joints
     Synovitis and inflammation of the capsule

3. Brain
   (i)   Sydenham's chorea
   (ii) Acute meningo-encephalitis
4. Skin
   (i)   Subcutaneous nodules
   (ii)   Erythema nodosum
   (iii) Erythema marginatum
   (iv)   Erythema multiforme
   (v)   Petechiae
   (vi)   Urticaria
   (vii) Livedo reticularis
5. Lungs
   Acute pneumonitis
6. Arteries
   Acute fibrinoid arteritis affecting coronary, cerebral, renal and
   mesenteric vessels

F. Infective endocarditis
Infecting organisms
1. *Streptococcus viridans*
2. Staphylococci
3. Enterococci *(Streptococcus faecalis)*
4. Brucellae
5. Haemophilus group
6. *Coxiella burnettii*
7. *Candida albicans*
8. *Histoplasma capsulatum*
9. *Aspergillus fumigatus*
10. *Cryptococcus neoformans*
Predisposing lesions
1. Valves previously damaged by rheumatic fever
2. Congenital valvular abnormalities e.g. bicuspid aortic valve
3. Interstitial valvulitis due to stress, hypersensitivity reactions,
   exposure to cold or high altitudes
4. ? Valvular endocarditis resulting from virus infections
Mechanism
1. Development of bland, fibrin-platelet thrombi on distorted or
   inflamed endocardium
2. Seeding of these small vegetations by organisms from the
   blood stream
3. Further fibrin deposition and proliferation of organisms give
   rise to larger, friable vegetations characteristic of infective
   endocarditis
Lesions of infective endocarditis
1. Features of infection and toxaemia
   (i)   Weight loss
   (ii)   Anaemia
   (iii) *Café au lait* skin pigmentation
   (iv)   Splenomegaly

2. Embolic features
   (i) Infarcts—brain, kidney, spleen
   (ii) Splinter haemorrhages
   (iii) Metastatic abscesses
   (iv) Mycotic aneurysms
3. Immune-complex deposition
   (i) Kidney lesions
      a. Focal glomerulonephritis ('embolic nephritis')
      b. Diffuse proliferative glomerulonephritis
   (ii) Brain
      a. Focal encephalitis
      b. Cerebral arteritis
   (iii) 'Microembolic' lesions
      a. Petechial rash
      b. Osler's nodes
      c. Roth's spots in the retina
      d. Retinal haemorrhage
      e. Nodular haemorrhagic lesions on palms and soles

Causes of death
1. Acute valve perforation
2. Embolism
3. Ruptured mycotic aneurysm
4. Renal failure—diffuse glomerulonephritis

G. Ischaemic heart disease
Aetiology
1. Coronary atherosclerosis alone or complicated by
   (i) Thrombosis
   (ii) Haemorrhage into a plaque
   (iii) Rupture of a plaque
2. Narrowing of the coronary ostia due to
   (i) Atherosclerosis
   (ii) Syphilitic aortitis
   (iii) Dissecting aneurysms
3. Coronary arteritis
4. Embolism
5. Trauma
6. Thrombotic diseases
7. Congenital abnormalities of the arteries
8. Irradiation

Types
1. Chronic ischaemic fibrosis
2. Infarction

Sequence of events in myocardial infarction

6—12 h —fibres show degenerative changes
        (i) Increased eosinophilia
        (ii) Swelling

12 h   —polymorphs appear

18 – 24 h—area paler than normal

48 h   —area outlined by a hyperaemic border, fibres become coagulated, and nuclear pyknosis increases

4 – 10 days—muscle becomes yellow and necrotic (myomalacia cordis) and there is increasing granulation tissue formation

12 days —collagen appears

3 weeks —infarct totally replaced by granulation tissue

3 months—shrunken scar

Complications
1. Fibrinous or haemorrhagic pericarditis
2. Mural thrombosis and embolism
3. Rupture giving cardiac tamponade
4. Cardiac aneurysm
5. Conduction defects
6. Cardiac failure

H. Tumours
1. Benign
   - (i) Atrial myxoma
   - (ii) Congenital rhabdomyoma (hamartoma)
2. Malignant (all very rare)
   - (i) Undifferentiated spindle-cell sarcoma
   - (ii) Rhabdomyosarcoma
   - (iii) Fibrosarcoma

ARTERIES

A. Arteriosclerosis and atherosclerosis (*see* p. 74)

B. Arteritis
1. Rheumatic fever
2. Rheumatoid disease
3. Ankylosing spondylitis
4. SLE
5. Polyarteritis nodosa
6. Wegener's granulomatosis
7. Thromboangiitis obliterans
8. Takayashu's disease
9. Giant-cell temporal arteritis
10. Infective causes
    - (i) Syphilis
    - (ii) Tuberculosis

11. Allergic vasculitis
    (i)   Visceral
          a. Appendix
          b. Gall-bladder
          c. Breast
          d. Urinary bladder
    (ii) Skin
          a. Erythema nodosum
          b. Erythema induratum
          c. Drug reactions
          d. Weber-Christian disease
          e. Nodular vasculitis

FURTHER READING

Hudson, R.E.B. (1970) *Cardiovascular Pathology*. London: Arnold.
Olsen, E.G.J. (1975) Cardiovascular system. In *Recent Advances in Pathology*, 9, ed. Harrison, C.V. & Weinbren, K. Edinburgh: Churchill Livingstone.
Symmers, W. St C. (Ed.) (1976) Cardiovascular system. *Systemic Pathology*, 2nd edn. Vol. 1. Edinburgh: Churchill Livingstone.

Respiratory system

NOSE AND NASAL SINUSES
A. Congenital
1. Choanal stenosis or atresia
2. Involvement in cleft palate
3. Saddle nose in hypertelorism

B. Inflammation
1. Acute rhinitis
   - (i) Common cold
   - (ii) Allergic
   - (iii) Measles
   - (iv) Irritant fumes
   - (v) Diphtheria
2. Acute sinusitis—non-specific, bacterial
3. Chronic hypertrophic rhinitis
4. Chronic atrophic rhinitis
   - (i) Simple atrophy
   - (ii) Ozaena
5. Chronic specific infections of the nose
   - (i) Tuberculosis
   - (ii) Leprosy
   - (iii) Syphilis
   - (iv) Scleroma
   - (v) Fungal infections
     - a. Candidiasis
     - b. Aspergillosis
     - c. Phycomycosis
     - d. Rhinosporidiosis
     - e. S. American blastomycosis
   - (vi) Leishmaniasis
6. 'Midline lethal granuloma'
   Types
   - (i) Wegener's granuloma
   - (ii) Primary lymphoma of the nose
   - (iii) Necrosis with atypical cellular exudate (probably histiocytic lymphoma)

C. Nasal polyps
1. Allergic
   - (i) Allergic rhinitis
   - (ii) Vasomotor rhinitis
2. Non-allergic including antro-choanal polyps

181

D. Tumours
1. Epithelial
   (i) Squamous papilloma
   (ii) Transitional-type ('inverted') papilloma
   (iii) Keratoacanthoma
   (iv) Adenoma arising from mucous glands
   (v) Carcinoma
      a. Squamous
      b. Transitional-type
      c. Adenocarcinoma
      d. Anaplastic
   (vi) Malignant melanoma
2. Vascular
   (i) Capillary haemangioma
   (ii) Juvenile angiofibroma
   (iii) Haemangiopericytoma
   (iv) Haemangioendothelioma (Angiosarcoma)
3. Lymphoid tissue
   (i) Lymphoma especially diffuse histiocytic type
   (ii) Myeloma
4. Neurogenic
   (i) Neurilemmoma
   (ii) Neurofibroma
   (iii) Nasal 'glioma' (ectopic glial tissue)
   (iv) Olfactory neuroblastoma
5. Bone and connective tissues
   (i) Osteoma
   (ii) Chondroma
   (iii) Ossifying fibroma
   (iv) Fibrosarcoma
   (v) Chondrosarcoma
   (vi) Osteogenic sarcoma

E. Tumours of the naso-pharynx
1. Benign
   (i) Transitional-type papilloma
   (ii) Adenoma
   (iii) Cavernous haemangioma
   (iv) Juvenile angiofibroma
2. Malignant
   (i) Carcinomas
      a. Anaplastic carcinoma including 'lymphoepithelioma'
      b. Squamous carcinoma
      c. Transitional-type carcinoma
      d. Adenocarcinoma
   (ii) Lymphoma and myeloma
   (iii) Sarcomas
      a. Rhabdomyosarcoma
      b. Fibrosarcoma
      c. Chondrosarcoma
   (iv) Chordoma arising from base of skull

LARYNX

A. Congenital
1. Laryngeal web
2. Stenosis
3. Laryngocele

B. Inflammation
1. Acute laryngitis (bacterial and viral)
2. Acute epiglottitis (*Haemophilus influenzae* type B)
3. Chronic laryngitis
   - (i) Non-specific
   - (ii) Tuberculosis
   - (iii) Syphilis
   - (iv) Fungal infections
   - (v) Scleroma
   - (vi) Leprosy

C. Polyps, cysts and benign tumours
1. Vocal cord polyps (Singer's nodes)
2. Cysts
   - (i) Mucus retention cysts
   - (ii) Epidermoid cysts
   - (iii) Branchial cysts
3. Benign tumours
   - (i) Juvenile papillomatosis
   - (ii) Adult papilloma
   - (iii) Adenoma of sero-mucinous glands
   - (iv) Papillary cystadenoma
   - (v) Chondroma
   - (vi) Neurogenic tumours
   - (vii) Lipoma
   - (viii) Granular cell myoblastoma

D. Pre-malignant and malignant lesions
1. 'Keratosis'
   Keratinisation and epithelial hyperplasia with or without dysplasia
2. Carcinoma-in-situ
3. Invasive carcinoma

Sites
(i)   Supraglottic
(ii)   Glottic—vocal cords and the commissures. This is the most frequent site and carries the best prognosis
(iii) Subglottic
(iv)   Transglottic—extensive tumours with a poor prognosis
Microscopic appearances
(i)   Squamous
(ii)   Anaplastic
(iii) Spindle-cell
(iv)   Verrucous squamous type
(v)   Adenocarcinoma
4. Sarcoma
(i)   Fibrosarcoma
(ii)   Chondrosarcoma

TRACHEA, BRONCHI AND LUNGS

A. Congenital
1. Agenesis of one lung
2. Hypoplasia of one or both lungs
3. Bronchogenic cystic disease of the lung
    (i)   Multiple
    (ii)   Single-pneumatocele
4. Cystic adenomatoid malformation
5. Accessory lobes
    (i)   Azygos
    (ii)   Cardiac
6. Absence of bronchial connections—sequestration
7. Abnormalities of the pulmonary arteries
8. Tracheo-oesophageal fistula

B. Inflammation of trachea and bronchi
1. Acute laryngo-tracheo-bronchitis
    (i)   Bacterial/viral
    (ii)   Atmospheric pollution
    (iii) Allergic
2. Chronic bronchitis
    'Expectoration of sputum on most days for three months or more, for at least two years.'
    Types
    (i)   Simple—only hypersecretion of mucus
    (ii)   Obstructive—where the hypersecretion is combined with airways obstruction
    Aetiology
    (i)   Smoking
    (ii)   Atmospheric pollution
    (iii) Persistent or recurrent infection, especially Haemophilus influenza
    (iv)   Familial predisposition

Gross features
(i)   Muco-purulent secretion
(ii) Symmetrical mild dilatation of bronchi
(iii) Prominent mucous glands which elevate the mucosa
(iv) Frequently associated with emphysema

Microscopic appearances
(i)   Bronchial epithelium
   a. Goblet-cell hyperplasia
   b. Variable squamous metaplasia
(ii) Bronchial sero-mucinous glands
   a. Hypertrophy
   b. Increased proportion of mucous to serous acini
   c. Gland to wall-thickness ratio (Reid index) increased
(iii) Submucosa
   Chronic inflammatory cell infiltration

Effects
(i)   Progressive dyspnoea
(ii) Cor pulmonale
(iii) Cardiac failure
(iv) Respiratory failure
   a. Hypercapnia
   b. Hypoxaemia

3. Bronchiectasis
   Dilatation of bronchi

Aetiology
(i)   Inflammatory disease of bronchial walls
   a. Unresolved pneumonia
   b. Pneumococcal bronchopneumonia
   c. Whooping cough
   d. Influenza
   e Measles
   f. Complicating chronic sinusitis
(ii) Extrinsic pressure on bronchi
   a. Lymph node enlargement e.g. primary tuberculosis
   b. Tumours
(iii) Intra-luminal obstruction
   a. Tenacious mucus in mucoviscidosis
   b. Foreign bodies
   c. Adenoma/carcinoma
   d. Pus and/or fibrinous exudates

Complications
(i)   Lung abscess
(ii) Empyema thoracis
(iii) Pyaemia—metastatic abscesses
(iv) Pulmonary fibrosis
(v)   Cor pulmonale and cardiac failure
(vi) Secondary amyloidosis

4. Bronchial asthma
Types
(i) Extrinsic
   a. Atopic asthma, Type I hypersensitivity to exogenous allergens
   b. Non-atopic, Type 3 hypersensitivity mediated by circulating precipitins
(ii) Intrinsic—attacks provoked by a wide variety of stimuli such as anxiety, infection etc.
(iii) Mixed type
Gross features
(i) Tenacious mucus plugs
(ii) Over-distension of lungs
(iii) Desquamation of epithelium
(iv) Sputum—Curschmann's spirals
   Charcot-Leyden crystals
Microscopic features in the bronchi
(i) Lumen filled with basophilic secretion
(ii) Eosinophils and desquamated epithelium in these plugs
(iii) Submucosal oedema
(iv) Infiltration by lymphocytes and eosinophils
(v) Serous acini increased relative to mucous acini
(vi) Muscular hypertrophy
Complications
(i) Recurrent pneumonia
(ii) Chronic bronchitis
(iii) Status asthmaticus
(iv) Pulmonary collapse

C. Acute pulmonary infections
1. Lung abscess
   (i) Inhalation of infected material, e.g. food, blood clot, teeth, etc.
   (ii) Complicating pneumonia/bronchiectasis
   (iii) Following bronchial obstruction especially due to carcinoma
   (iv) Pyaemic (secondary) abscesses
   Complications
   (i) Scarring and deformity of the lung
   (ii) Empyema
   (iii) Broncho-pleural fistula
   (iv) Pyaemia
2. Acute bacterial pneumonia
   (i) Lobar pneumonia
      Causes
      a. Pneumococci, Types I, II, VII and II account for 90 – 95% of cases
      b. Klebsiella
      c. Staphylococci
      d. Streptococci
      e. H. influenza

Stages
a. Congestion
b. Red hepatisation
c. Grey hepatisation
d. Resolution
Complications
a. Empyema
b. Suppurative pericarditis
c. Metastatic abscesses
d. Acute endocarditis
e. Meningitis
f. Arthritis
g. Peritonitis
(ii) Bronchopneumonia (lobular)
Causes
a. Pneumococci
b. H. influenza
c. Staphylococci
d. Streptococci
e. Klebsiella
f. Yersinia pestis (plague)
g. Anthrax ('wool-sorter's disease')
Complications
a. 'Carnification'—organisation of exudate
b. Pulmonary fibrosis—scarring in areas destroyed by suppuration
c. Bronchiectasis
d. Lung abscess
e. Empyema
f. Pericarditis
g. Metastatic abscesses
3. Viral pneumonia
Causes
a. Influenza
b. Adenoviruses
c. Rhinoviruses
d. Corona viruses
e. Measles
f. Cytomegalic inclusion
4. Chlamydiae (Bedsonia)
a. Psittacosis
b. Ornithosis
5. 'Primary atypical pneumonia'
Causes
a. Mycoplasma pneumoniae (majority of cases)
b. Influenza viruses
c. Respiratory syncitial virus
d. Rhinoviruses
e. Coxsackie
f. ECHO virus   rare
6. Rickettsial pneumonia—*Coxiella burnettii*

D. Chronic pulmonary infections
1. Tuberculosis (see p. 56)
2. Actinomycosis
3. Nocardiosis
4. Fungal infections
   (i) Aspergillosis
   (ii) Candidiasis
   (iii) Phycomycosis
   (iv) Cryptococcosis
   (v) Blastomycosis
   (vi) Histoplasmosis
   (vii) Torulopsis glabrata
5. Protozoan infections
   (i) Pneumocystis carinii
   (ii) Amoebiasis
6. Metazoan infections
   (i) Schistosomiasis
   (ii) Paragonimiasis
   (iii) Ascariasis
   (iv) Hydatid disease

E. Diffuse pulmonary fibrosis
Widespread fibrosis may be caused by
1. Organising pneumonia, e.g. influenza
2. Chronic pulmonary oedema
3. Pneumoconiosis
   (i) Coal workers'
      a. Simple pneumoconiosis
      b. Progressive massive fibrosis
      c. Caplan's type (with rheumatoid arthritis)
   (ii) Silicosis
   (iii) Asbestosis—
      also gives rise to
      a. Pleural thickening
      b. Bronchial carcinoma
      c. Mesothelioma
   (iv) Berylliosis
   (v) Bauxite lung
4. Sarcoidosis
5. Extrinsic allergic alveolitis (see p. 40)
6. Diffuse fibrosing alveolitis
   Features
   (i) Desquamation into alveoli of type 2 pneumocytes
      (? Desquamative Interstitial Pneumonia)
   (ii) Mural fibrosis and lymphocytic infiltration
7. Eosinophil granuloma
8. Rheumatoid disease
9. Wegener's granulomatosis
10. Giant-cell interstitial pneumonia
11. Lymphocytic interstitial pneumonia
12. Hypersensitivity to drugs—nitrofurantoin, salazopyrine
13. Cytotoxic damage—busulphan, hexamethonium, bleomycin

F. Pulmonary emphysema
Classification
1. Interstitial emphysema—the presence of air in the interstitial tissue of the lung
   Causes
   (i) Tearing of alveolar walls by excessive pressure
      a. Severe asthma
      b. Whooping cough
      c. Blast injury
      d. Intermittent positive-pressure ventilation
   (ii) Tearing of alveolar walls by direct trauma
      a. Fractured ribs
      b. Needle biopsy
2. Vesicular emphysema—an increase beyond the normal in air spaces distal to terminal bronchioles, that is the pulmonary acini.
   An acinus contains the respiratory bronchioles, alveolar ducts, and alveoli arising from one terminal bronchiole.
   (i) Centriacinar (centrilobular) emphysema
   Distensive type found in
      a. Urban dwellers
      b. Coal-miners
   Destructive types—more severe form in
      a. Chronic bronchitis
      b. Smoking
   (ii) Panacinar emphysema
   Distensive type
      a. Lobar emphysema of infancy and childhood
      b. Compensatory emphysema following collapse, agenesis, surgical removal
   Destructive type
      a. Chronic bronchitis and recurrent bronchopneumonia
      b. α-1—antitrypsin deficiency
      c. Inhalation of cadmium fumes (? in cigarette smoke)
   (iii) Paraseptal (periacinar) emphysema
      ? results from inflammation
   (iv) Irregular emphysema
      This does not affect the acini in a uniform manner.
   Occurence
      a. relation to scars
      b. giant bullous emphysema
      c. acute tension cysts of infancy

G. Mechanical disorders
1. Pulmonary atelectasis
   A failure of full expansion of the lungs after birth
   Causes
   (i) Bronchial obstruction
      a. Viscid mucus
      b. Liquor amnii
   (ii) In association with hyaline membrane disease
   (iii) Brain damage involving the respiratory centre

2. Lung collapse (after full aeration)
   Causes
   (i)   Obstruction of the bronchial lumen
         a. Mucus in asthma, mucoviscidosis
         b. Aspirated material
         c. After anaesthesia/operations
         d. Foreign bodies
   (ii) Extreme narrowing of a bronchus
         a. Carcinoma
         b. Inflammatory fibrosis
   (iii) External pressure on a bronchus
         a. Enlarged lymph gland
         b. Aortic aneurysm
         c. Tumour
   (iv) Pressure on the lung
         a. Pneumothorax
         b. Pleural effusion
         c. G-forces in aircrew

H. Vascular disorders
   1. Pulmonary oedema
      Causes
      (i)   Left ventricular failure
      (ii)   Inflammatory oedema
             a. Infection
                Bacterial/viral pneumonias etc
             b. Hypersensitivity reactions
                Bee stings, iodine, nitrofurantoin
      (iii) Toxic injury
             a. Irritant fumes
                Smoke, ammonia, sulphur dioxide
             b. Drugs—Busulphan, Hexamethonium
             c. Uraemia
      (iv)   Raised intracranial pressure
      (v)   Trauma
             a. Direct injury to the chest
             b. Blast injury
             c. Thoracic surgery
      (vi)   Hypoproteinaemia, as in
             a. Renal failure
             b. Hepatic failure
             c. Malabsorption
      (vii) Hypoxia—acute high-altitude oedema
      (viii) Lymphatic obstruction—mainly carcinomatous

I. Benign tumours

1. Epithelial
   - (i) Adenoma of mucous gland origin
   - (ii) Papilloma
   - (iii) Paraganglionoma
2. Connective tissues
   - (i) Lipoma
   - (ii) Fibroma
   - (iii) Angioma and sclerosing angioma
   - (iv) Chondroma
   - (v) Pseudolymphoma
   - (vi) Neurofibroma
3. Mixed tumour—chondroadenoma (hamartoma)

J. Malignant tumours

1. Bronchial carcinoma

   Aetiology
   - (i) Cigarette smoking (?)
   - (ii) Atmospheric pollution (?)
   - (iii) Asbestosis
   - (iv) Arsenic exposure
   - (v) Workers with nickel, haematite and chromates

   Types
   - (i) Squamous carcinoma (via squamous metaplasia)
   - (ii) Small cell anaplastic carcinoma – oat cell carcinoma probably originating from bronchial APUD cells
   - (iii) Adenocarcinoma
     - a. Bronchial adenocarcinoma
     - b. Bronchiolo-alveolar carcinoma
   - (iv) Large cell carcinoma
     - a. Anaplastic solid large-cell carcinomas
     - b. 'Clear-cell' carcinoma
     - c. Giant-cell carcinoma

   Spread
   - (i) Local
   - (ii) Lymphatic—lymphangitis carcinomatosa
   - (iii) Blood
     - a. Liver
     - b. Adrenals
     - c. Brain
     - d. Skeleton
     - e. Kidneys

2. Bronchial carcinoid tumour
    May give rise to carcinoid syndrome and endocardial fibrosis
    of the left side of the heart
3. Malignant tumours of mucous glands
    (i)   Adenoid cystic carcinoma (cribriform adenocarcinoma)
    (ii)   Mucoepidermoid tumour
4. Carcinosarcomas
    (i)   'True' type
    (ii)   Embryonal type—pulmonary blastoma
5. Sarcomas
    (i)   Leiomyosarcoma
    (ii)   Fibrosarcoma
    (iii) Neurofibrosarcoma
    (iv)   Rhabdomyosarcoma
6. Malignant lymphomas

FURTHER READING

Batsakis, J.G. (1974) *Tumors of the Head and Neck.* Baltimore:
    Williams & Wilkins.
Spencer, H. (1977) *Pathology of the Lung,* 3rd edn. Oxford:
    Pergamon Press.
Symmers, W. St C. (Ed.) (1976) Respiratory system. *Systemic
    Pathology,* 2nd edn., Vol. 1. Edinburgh: Churchill Livingstone.

Genito-urinary system

KIDNEY

A. Congenital and inherited malformations
1. Agenesis
2. Hypoplasia
3. Heterotopic sites, e.g. pelvic
4. Fusion—horseshoe kidney
5. Cysts
   (i) Polycystic kidney
   a. Infantile type
   b. Adult type
   (ii) Medullary cysts
   a. Medullary cystic disease (nephronophthisis)
   b. Medullary sponge kidney
   (iii) Cortical cysts
   a. 'Pluricystic kidney' associated with multiple malformation syndromes, e.g. Down's, Turner's, Von Hippel-Lindau, etc.
   b. Congenital nephrotic syndrome
   (iv) (Cystic) Renal dysplasia

B. Inflammatory disorders (mainly affecting the interstitium)

1. *Acute pyelonephritis*
Acute bacterial infection of the kidney and renal pelvis, usually resulting from ascending infection of the urinary tract, but some cases may result from haematogenous or lymphatic spread.
Pathogenesis
Ascending infection usually follows bacterial contamination of the urine in the bladder with or without true infection of the bladder wall—cystitis.
   Predisposing factors
   (i) Obstruction, of which the major causes are
   a. Malformations of the tract in childhood
   b. Pregnancy
   c. Prostatic hyperplasia and uterine prolapse in the elderly
   (ii) Ureteric reflux
   (iii) Catheterisation
   (iv) Diabetes mellitus
   Pathological features
   (i) Kidney is swollen and hyperaemic
   (ii) Surface studded with small abscesses
   (iii) Scattered, rounded or linear abscesses in the cortex and medulla
   (iv) Polymorphs in tubules and interstitium

Complications
(i)   Renal carbuncle
(ii) Peri-nephric abscess
(iii) Renal papillary necrosis
(iv) Acute renal failure
(v)   Pyonephrosis
(vi) Chronic pyelonephritis

2. *Chronic pyelonephritis*
Chronic inflammation and fibrosis associated with persistent infection or initiated by infection but becoming self-perpetuating
Pathological features
(i)   Granular, shrunken kidneys
(ii) Cortical scarring
(iii) Deformity of the pelvi-calyceal system
Microscopic
(iv) Tubular atrophy
(v)   Interstitial fibrosis
(vi) Periglomerular fibrosis
(vii) Glomerular hyalinisation
Complications
(i)   Hypertension
(ii) Chronic renal failure

3. *Tuberculosis*
(i)   Miliary
(ii) Fibro-caseous, nodular tuberculosis
(iii) Tuberculous 'pyonephrosis'

C. Glomerular disorders
1. *Proliferative glomerulonephritis*
(i)   Diffuse proliferative GN
      Results from deposition of immune complexes formed in response to
      a. Streptococcal infection
      Rare causes are
      b. Sub-acute bacterial endocarditis
      c. Straphylococcal bacteraemia
      d. Virus infections; mumps, chicken-pox, measles
      e. Viral hepatitis antigen
      Microscopic features
      a. Proliferation of endothelial and mesangial cells
      b. Polymorph exudation
      c. Subepithelial deposits of IgG, C_3 etc. on immunofluorescence
(ii) Rapidly progressive proliferative GN
      Aetiology
      a. Idiopathic
      b. Post-streptococcal
      c. Goodpasture's syndrome
      d. Henoch-Schönlein syndrome
      e. Lupus glomerulonephritis

Pathological features
a. Proliferation of epithelial cells lining Bowman's capsule
b. Hypercellularity of glomerular tuft
Prognosis: very poor

(iii) Mesangial proliferative GN
Aetiology
a. Idiopathic
b. Healing phase of post-streptococcal GN
Pathology
Hypercellularity of the central or axial regions due to mesangial cell proliferation
Prognosis: generally good

(iv) Mesangiocapillary
(formerly membrano-proliferative)
Aetiology: idiopathic
Pathological features
a. Mesangial cell proliferation
b. Thickening of the glomerular basement membrane (GBM)
c. Increase in mesangial connective tissue and deposition of fibrils internal to the GBM
d. Exaggerated lobular pattern
e. Hypocomplementaemia
Prognosis: usually slowly progressive

(v) Focal proliferative GN
Focal (random) and segmental involvement of glomeruli with IgA deposits (IgA nephropathy) or associated with systemic diseases:
a. Bacterial endocarditis ('focal embolic')
b. SLE
c. Drug reactions (hypersensitivity type)
d. Polyarteritis nodosa
e. Goodpasture's syndrome
f. Henoch-Schönlein syndrome
g. Wegener's granulomatosis

2. *Membranous nephropathy*
Aetiology: idiopathic (? immune disorder)
Rare causes
(ii) Drug hypersensitivity, particularly gold
(iii) Secondary and congenital syphilis
(iv) Quartan malaria
(v) Extra-renal malignancy
(vi) SLE
Pathological features
(i) Diffuse thickening of the GBM with 'spike' formation
(ii) Deposits of immunoglobulin and complement beneath epithelium
(iii) The epithelial podocytes lose their foot processes
(iv) Progressive sclerosis of glomeruli
Prognosis: usually presents with nephrotic syndrome and progresses slowly to renal failure in 5 – 10 years

3. Minimal change disease (lipoid nephrosis)
This is the most common cause of the nephrotic syndrome in childhood

Aetiology
? hypersensitivity to drugs, insect stings, toxins, pollens, food, mediated by IgE antibody
Pathological features
(i) Fusion of epithelial foot processes (EM)
(ii) Fat droplets in the tubular epithelium
Prognosis: excellent when treated with diuretics, corticosteroids or cytotoxics, and removal of allergen if identifiable

4. Focal glomerulosclerosis
Hyaline thickening of mesangial regions and capillary loops of focal and segmental distribution, usually presenting as the nephrotic syndrome
Poor response to treatment

5. Chronic glomerulonephritis
The end result of a variety of progressive destructive lesions

Aetiology. The main causes are
(i)   Progressive diffuse proliferative GN
(ii) Later stages of membranous nephropathy
(iii) Idiopathic
Pathological features
(i)   Contracted kidneys
(ii) Hyaline fibrosis of glomeruli
(iii) Secondary tubular atrophy
(iv) Interstitial fibrosis
(v)   Associated vascular changes of hypertension
Prognosis: chronic renal failure and death

Pathological basis of the clinical syndromes
(i)   Acute nephritis syndrome
    a. Diffuse proliferative GN
    b. Rapidly progressive GN
    c. Mesangio-capillary GN
    d. SLE
    e. Polyarteritis nodosa
    f. Henoch-Schönlein syndrome
    g. IgA nephropathy
    h. Hereditary nephritis
(ii) Nephrotic syndrome
    a. Minimal change
    b. Membranous nephropathy
    c. Proliferative GN
    d. Focal glomerulosclerosis
    e. Amyloidosis
    f. Diabetes mellitus
    g. SLE
    h. Renal vein thrombosis
    i. Congenital nephrotic syndrome

    (iii) Acute renal failure
- a. Acute tubular necrosis
- b. Rapidly progressive GN
- c. Diffuse proliferative GN
- d. Severe acute pyelonephritis
- e. Malignant hypertension
- f. Polyarteritis nodosa
- g. SLE
- h. Eclampsia
- i. Hypercalcaemia
- j. Haemolytic-uraemic syndrome

    (iv) Chronic renal failure
- a. Chronic glomerulonephritis
- b. Chronic pyelonephritis
- c. Hypertensive nephrosclerosis
- d. Diabetes mellitus

    (v) Painless haematuria
- a. Minimal change
- b. Mesangial proliferative GN
- c. Progressive proliferative GN
- d. Chronic pyelonephritis
- e. Hydronephrosis
- f. Calculus
- g. Tumours
- h. Benign recurrent haematuria

D. Tubular disorders

1. *Acute tubular necrosis*

    (i) Nephrotoxic
- a. Heavy metals
- b. Organic solvents
- c. Ethylene glycol
- d. Mushroom poisoning

    (ii) Ischaemic
The causes are those of 'shock'

Pathological features

    (i) Kidneys are swollen and pale

    (ii) Tubular epithelial necrosis, with desquamation of cells forming casts

    (iii) Calcium oxalate crystals in the lumen in some cases

    (iv) Rupture of the tubular basement membrane—tubulorrhexis

    (v) Regeneration of epithelium in later stages

2. *Myeloma kidney*

3. *Bile nephrosis*

4. *Glycogen accumulation*

    (i) Diabetes mellitus

    (ii) Glycogenoses

5. *Tubular vacuolation*

    (i) Hypokalaemia

    (ii) Administration of hypertonic solutions

6. *Disorders of tubular function*
    (i)   Defects in transport mechanisms
         a. Renal glycosuria
         b. Phosphaturia
         c. Renal tubular acidosis
         d. Familial phospho-gluco-aminoaciduria
         e. Cystinuria
         f. Hartnup disease
         g. Glycine-iminoaciduria
         h. Glycinuria
    (ii) Abnormal tubular response to hormones
         a. Nephrogenic diabetes insipidus
         b. Pseudohypoparathyroidism
         c. Pseudohypoaldosteronism
         d. Pseudohyperaldosteronism

E. Urinary calculi and nephrocalcinosis

Calculi
Calculi are composed of amorphous urinary crystalloids bound by a mucoprotein matrix. They may be found anywhere in the urinary tract but most are formed in the calyces and renal pelvis. The major crystalloids are:
1. Uric acid
2. Urates
3. Oxalates
4. Calcium or magnesium phosphate

Pathogenesis
1. Increased concentration of crystalloids in the urine resulting from:
    (i)   Reduced urine volume as in dehydration
    (ii) Increased excretion of crystalloids
         a. Hypercalciuria
         b. Cystinuria
         c. Gout—(uric acid excess)
2. Factors favouring the precipitation of crystalloids from 'normal' urine
    (i)   Stasis
    (ii) Infection. Organisms may split urea and produce alkalinity of the urine which favours the formation of magnesium-ammonium phosphate
    (iii) Foreign bodies, clumps of bacteria, desquamated epithelial cells, act as a nidus for crystallisation
    (iv) Deficiency of stabilising factors such as citrate, colloids, amino acids

Effects
1. Obstruction—hydronephrosis
2. Chronic infection—pyelonephritis

Nephrocalcinosis
  Aetiology
  1. Hyperparathyroidism
  2. Malignancy
     (i) Hypercalcaemia due to osteolytic deposits
     (ii) Secretion of parathormone-like hormone by tumour cells
  3. Paget's disease of bone particularly during immobilisation
  4. Sarcoidosis
  5. Vitamin D excess
  6. Milk-alkali syndrome
  7. Renal tubular acidosis
  8. Idiopathic hypercalcaemia of infancy
  9. Hyperoxaluria
  10. Hyperthyroidism
  11. Hypothyroidism in infants

F. Vascular disorders
  1. Benign nephrosclerosis in essential hypertension
  2. Malignant nephrosclerosis
  3. Senile arteriosclerotic disease
  4. Infarction
     (i) Arterial embolism
        a. Atrial or mural thrombosis in the heart
        b. Thrombus from the aorta
        c. Atherosclerotic debris from ruptured plaque
     (ii) Arterial thrombosis
        a. Superimposed on atherosclerosis
        b. Aortic thrombosis
        c. Polyarteritis nodosa
     (iii) Involvement of renal ostia by aneurysm
     (iv) Sudden venous occlusion resulting from
          thrombophlebitis
  5. Acute cortical necrosis resulting from DIC in various forms of
     shock.

G. Tumours

  1. *Benign*
     (i) Cortical adenoma
     (ii) Fibroma
     (iii) Haemangioma
     (iv) Angiolipomyoma

  2. *Malignant*
     (i) Adenocarcinoma
        a. Solid-cell type ⎱ often found in the
        b. Clear-cell type ⎰ same tumour
     (ii) Nephroblastoma (Wilm's tumour)
     (iii) Sarcomas (very rare)
     (iv) Transitional cell carcinoma of the renal pelvis

BLADDER
A. Congenital
1. Diverticula
2. Ectopia vesicae
3. Persistent urachus

B. Inflammations
1. Acute cystitis
2. Chronic cystitis
3. Special forms of cystitis
   - (i)   Follicular
   - (ii)   Encrusted—phosphates
   - (iii)   Bullous
   - (iv)   Interstitial
   - (v)   Cystitis cystica
   - (vi)   Tuberculous
   - (vii)   Malakoplakia
   - (viii) Irradiation
   - (ix)   Schistosomiasis (haematobium)

C. Tumours
1. Transitional cell papilloma
2. Transitional cell carcinoma
3. Squamous carcinoma
4. Adenocarcinoma
5. Sarcomas—rhabdomyosarcoma

PROSTATE
A. Inflammations
1. Non-specific prostatitis
   - (i)   Acute
   - (ii)   Chronic
   - (iii)   Granulomatous
2. Tuberculous prostatitis
3. Eosinophilic (allergic) prostatitis

B. Nodular hyperplasia
Types of nodule
1. Fibromyoadenomatous
2. Fibroadenomatous
3. Stromal (fibrous)
4. Fibrovascular—possibly resulting from previous infarction or foci of inflammation
5. Muscular

Additional features
1. Focal inflammation—acute or chronic
2. Corpora amylacea
3. Calculi
4. Cystic degeneration
5. Infarcts
6. Squamous metaplasia/hyperplasia of the peri-urethral glands

C. Carcinoma
Aetiological factors
(i)   Age—rare under 50
(ii) Hormones
    a. ? steroid imbalance
    b. ? altered sensitivity of prostatic epithelium
(iii) Race—low incidence in Orientals
Histological types
(i)   Adenocarcinoma
(ii) Anaplastic
(iii) Squamous carcinoma arising from metaplastic
    epithelium in ducts
Behavioural types
(i)   Clinical prostatic cancer—where the disease is
    producing symptoms
(ii) Latent cancer—small foci of carcinoma found
    incidentally at prostatectomy or autopsy and have not
    yet spread
(iii) Occult cancer—the appearance of metastases whilst the
    primary remains covert
Stages
A =Occult carcinoma
B =Nodule of carcinoma confined within the prostatic
    capsule
C =Carcinoma has spread outside the capsule with
    extension into surrounding structures, or confined
    within the capsule but with elevated serum acid
    phosphatase
D =Demonstrable skeletal or extra-pelvic involvement
Spread
(i)   Direct: seminal vesicles, rectum, bladder
(ii) Lymphatic: iliac, para-aortic glands
(iii) Blood: bone, particularly the sacrum and vertebrae

TESTIS AND EPIDIDYMIS
A. Congenital
1. Undescended testis (cryptorchidism)
2. Absence of one or both testes
3. Fusion
4. Simple cysts
5. Ectopic testes

B. Inflammatory disorders
1. Non-specific epididymo-orchitis
2. Gonococcal epididymo-orchitis
3. Mumps orchitis
4. Tuberculosis (starts in epididymis)
5. Syphilis (starts in testis)
6. Granulomatous orchitis

C. Degenerative disorders
1. Atrophy
   Causes
   (i)   Increasing age—? ischaemic
   (ii)   Following orchitis
   (iii) Administration of anabolic steroids
   (iv)   Malnutrition
   (v)   Post-vasectomy
   (vi)   Hyperoestrogenic states
   (vii) Hypopituitarism
2. Hypoplasia
   (i)   Cryptorchidism
   (ii)   Klinefelter's syndrome

D. Vascular disorders
1. Torsion of the testis
2. Varicocoele (varicosity of the pampiniform plexus)

E. Tumours
1. Seminoma (40%)
   A malignant tumour of germ cells, mainly arising from
   spermatogonia but a small proportion are spermatocytic
   Spread
   (i)   Lymphatic: iliac and para-aortic lymph glands
   (ii)   Blood: late spread to lungs and liver
   Prognosis
   (i)   without lymph node involvement, 98% survival at 5
          years
   (ii)   with nodal involvement, 90% at 5 years
   (iii) with visceral metastases, 20% at 5 years
2. Teratoma differentiated (Teratoma)
   Cysts lined by a variety of mature epithelia, together with
   cartilage, bone, marrow, glia, etc.
3. Malignant teratoma intermediate (Teratocarcinoma)
   Tumour showing organoid differentiation and/or mature
   tissue with malignant areas elsewhere
4. Malignant teratoma undifferentiated (Embryonal carcinoma)
5. Malignant teratoma trophoblastic (Choriocarcinoma)
6. Interstitial cell tumour
   A tumour derived from Leydig cells which are often
   associated with endocrine effects such as gynaecomastia or
   sexual precosity in childhood. 10% are malignant.
7. Orchioblastoma
   Tumours of low-grade malignancy presenting in infancy and
   resembling a papillary adenocarcinoma
8. Carcinoma of the rete and appendix testis
9. Sertoli-cell tumour—very rare benign tumour
10. Tumours of the epididymis
    (i)   Adenomatoid tumour
    (ii)   Carcinoma

UTERUS

A. Congenital
1. Abnormal fusion of the Mullerian ducts
   (i) Double uterus
   (ii) Septate
   (iii) Bicornuate, etc.

B. Inflammations
1. Acute endometritis (pyometria)
2. Chronic endometritis
3. Tuberculous endometritis

C. Endometriosis
1. Uterine
   (i) Adenomyosis
   (ii) Stromal endometriosis
2. External
   Sites
   (i) Ovaries
   (ii) Fallopian tubes
   (iii) Rectovaginal septum
   (iv) Peritoneum
   (v) Umbilicus
   (vii) Rare sites—vulva, vagina, appendix, intestinal wall
   Effects
   (i) 'Chocolate' cyst formation
   (ii) Intra-pelvic haemorrhage
   (iii) Formation of adhesions

D. Effects of hormonal abnormalities
1. Delayed shedding
2. Oral contraceptive effects
   (i) Pseudo-decidual change (progesterone)
   (ii) Disparity between stromal and glandular appearances
3. Arias-Stella phenomenon
4. Cystic hyperplasia
   (i) Diffuse
   (ii) Polypoid
5. Atypical hyperplasia
6. Senile cystic atrophy

E. Tumours
1. Myometrium
    (i)   Leiomyoma (fibroid)
    (ii) Adenomyoma
    (iii) Angiomyoma
    (iv) Leiomyosarcoma
2. Endometrium
    (i)   Carcinoma
          Predisposing factors
          a. Atypical endometrial hyperplasia
          b. Ovarian stromal hyperplasia
          c. Granulosa-theca tumours of the ovary
          d. Stein-Leventhal syndrome
    The tumour is more common in nulliparous women.
          Histological types
          a. Adenocarcinoma, frequently with squamous
             metaplasia (adenoacanthoma)
          b. Adenosquamous, where there is a mixture of
             adenocarcinoma and malignant squamous
             elements—this has a worse prognosis
          Spread
          a. Direct to tubes and ovaries
          b. Lymphatic to iliac, inguinal, and para-aortic glands
          c. Blood spread is late—lungs, liver, adrenals and bone
    (ii) Stromal tumours
          a. Endolymphatic stromal myosis
          b. Stromal sarcoma

CERVIX
A. Inflammations
1. Acute cervicitis
2. Chronic cervicitis
    Features
    (i)   Chronic inflammatory cells with, in a few cases, follicle
          formation
    (ii) Inflammatory dysplasia of squamous epithelium with
          loss of glycogen
    (iii) Epidermidisation of endocervical-type glands
    (iv) Nabothian cysts

B. Tumours
1. Cervical polyp
   (i) Endocervical or mucous polyp
   (ii) Inflammatory polyp (granulation tissue)
2. Papillomata
   (i) Squamous papilloma
   (ii) Condyloma acuminata
3. Carcinoma
   Predisposing factors
   (i) Low social class
   (ii) Promiscuity, frequency of intercourse, early age of onset of sexual relations
   (iii) Chronic cervicitis
   (iv) Low incidence where male circumcision is practised
   Natural history
   (i) Chronic cervicitis
   (ii) Epithelial dysplasia
   (iii) Carcinoma-in-situ
   (iv) Invasive carcinoma
   Gross types
   (i) Fungating
   (ii) Ulcerated
   (iii) Infiltrative or indurated
   Histological types
   (i) Squamous carcinoma (95%)
   (ii) Adenocarcinoma
   (iii) Adenoacanthoma
   Staging
Stage O = Carcinoma-in-situ
Stage I = Invasive carcinoma confined to the cervix
Stage II = Carcinoma extends beyond the cervix but not to the pelvic wall or lower ⅓ of vagina
Stage III = Carcinoma extends to pelvic wall and/or the lower ⅓ of vagina
Stage IV = Extension beyond the true pelvis or involvement of mucosa of bladder or rectum
4. Mixed mesodermal tumour (Sarcoma botryoides)
   A malignant tumour composed of smooth muscle, fibrous and myxoid tissue, cartilage and bone. It occurs at all ages including childhood and may arise from cervix, vagina or uterus.

OVARY

Tumours	Benign	Malignant
1. Arising from coelomic epithelium	Mucinous cystadenoma	Mucinous cystadenocarcinoma
	Serous cystadenoma	Serous cystadenocarcinoma Endometrioid carcinoma Clear-cell carcinoma (Mesonephroma)
2. Connective tissue (stromal) origin	Fibroma	Fibrosarcoma
	Haemangioma	Angiosarcoma
3. Mixed epithelial and stromal tumours	Cystadenofibroma Brenner tumour	
4. Functioning tumours of sex cord—mesenchymal origin		Granulosa-theca-luteal tumours Arrhenoblastoma Hilus (Leydig) cell tumour
5. Germ-cell tumours (including teratoma)		Dysgerminoma
	Cystic teratoma (dermoid)	Malignant teratoma
		Chorioncarcinoma
6. Secondary tumours		from primary carcinoma in breast, gastrointestinal tract, uterus or other ovary

BREAST

A. Congenital
 1. Supernumerary nipples—polythelia
 2. Supernumerary breasts—polymastia

B. Inflammations
 1. Acute suppurative mastitis
 2. Breast abscess
 3. Mammary duct ectasia (plasma-cell mastitis)
 4. Fat necrosis
 5. Tuberculosis
 6. Silicone mastitis following cosmetic surgery

C. Mammary dysplasia

Syn: Cystic mastopathy
Fibrocystic disease

Microscopic features (found in various combinations)

1. Cyst formation (macro- or microcysts)
2. Inter- and intralobular fibrosis
3. Apocrine metaplasia
4. Epithelial proliferation (epitheliosis)
5. Ductular proliferation (adenosis)
6. Papillomatosis
7. Lobular sclerosis (sclerosing adenosis)

Occasionally, *sclerosing adenosis* is found as a solitary lesion. In some young women fibrosis is the dominant feature and is associated with premature involution. This form has been designated *fibrous disease of the breast*.

D. Tumours

Benign

1. Fibroadenoma
   (i) Intracanalicular
   (ii) Pericanalicular
2. Intraduct papilloma
3. Adenoma of the nipple
4. Lipoma
5. Fibroma, haemangioma, etc.

Intermediate
Giant fibroadenoma (cystosarcoma phylloides)

Malignant

1. Non-invasive carcinoma
   (i) Intraduct carcinoma
   (ii) Intralobular carcinoma
2. Invasive carcinoma
   (i) Scirrhous carcinoma and
   (ii) Medullary carcinoma, showing varying degrees of differentiation from well-formed tubules (adenocarcinoma) to undifferentiated (anaplastic) growths
   (iii) Papillary carcinoma
   (iv) Mucoid (colloid) carcinoma
   (v) Apocrine-type carcinoma
   (vi) Squamous carcinoma
   (vii) Adenoid-cystic carcinoma
3. Paget's disease of the nipple associated with underlying ductal carcinoma.

Spread of mammary carcinoma
1. Direct
   (i)   Skin—fungating growths
   (ii) Deep fascia
   (iii) Muscle
2. Lymphatic
   (i)   Axillary and internal mammary lymph glands
   (ii) Dermal lymphatics
   (iii) Widespread dissemination—mediastinal, abdominal,
         pelvic and inguinal glands
3. Serous cavities with effusions
   (i)   Pleura
   (ii) Pericardium
4. Blood stream
   (i)   Lungs
   (ii) Bone
   (iii) Adrenals
   (iv) Ovaries
   (v)   Kidneys
   (vi) Brain, etc.

Other malignant tumours of the breast
All are rare
1. Fibrosarcoma
2. Liposarcoma
3. Haemangiosarcoma
4. Lymphoma

FURTHER READING

Fox, H. & Langley, F.A. (Eds.) (1973) *Postgraduate Obstetrical and Gynaecological Pathology.* Oxford: Pergamon Press.

Fox, H. & Langley, F.A. (1976) *Tumours of the Ovary.* London: Heinemann.

Heptinstall, R.H. (1974) *Pathology of the Kidney,* 2nd edn. Boston: Little Brown.

Journal of Clinical Pathology (1976) The pathology of pregnancy. *Journal of Clinical Pathology,* Suppl. 10.

Meadows, R. (1973) *Renal Histopathology.* London: Oxford University Press.

Mostofi, F.K. & Price, E.B. (1973) Tumors of the male genital system. *Atlas of Tumor Pathology,* 2nd series, 3. Montvale, N.J.: A.F.I.P.S. Press.

Novak, E.R. & Woodruff, J.D. (1974) *Gynecologic and Obstetric Pathology,* 7th edn. Philadelphia: Saunders.

Pugh, R.C.B. (Ed.) (1976) *Pathology of the Testis.* Oxford: Blackwell.

Tighe, J.R. (1975) Diseases of the kidney. In *Recent Advances in Pathology,* 9, ed. Harrison, C.V. & Weinbren, K., p. 131. Edinburgh: Churchill Livingstone.

Williams, D.I. & Chisholm, G.D. (Ed.) (1976) *Scientific Foundations of Urology.* London: Heinemann.

Lymphoid tissue

A. Reactive lymphadenopathy
1. Acute reactions to infection characterised by
    (i)   Enlargement
    (ii) Sinus 'catarrh'
    (iii) Sinus histiocytosis
    (iv) Follicular hyperplasia
2. Suppurative/tuberculoid
    Aetiology
    (i)   Yersinia pseudotuberculosis
    (ii) Lymphogranuloma venereum
    (iii) Cat-scratch fever
    (iv) Coccidioidomycosis
3. Tuberculoid
    Aetiology
    (i)   Tuberculosis
    (ii) Sarcoidosis
    (iii) Sarcoid-like granulomata (see p. 000)
4. Pigment reactions
    (i)   Anthracosis
    (ii) Silicosis
    (iii) Dermatopathic lymphadenopathy
    (iv) Cholegranulomatous lymphadenopathy
5. Hodgkin's-like picture
    (i)   Early tuberculosis/sarcoidosis
    (ii) Toxoplasmosis
    (iii) Drug reactions, e.g. phenytoin
    (iv) Infectious mononucleosis
    (v)   Immunoblastic lymphadenopathy

B. Lymphoma
1. Hodgkin's disease
    Varieties (Rye classification)
    (i)   Nodular sclerosis
    (ii) Lymphocyte predominant
    (iii) Mixed cellularity
    (iv) Lymphocyte depleted

2. Non-Hodgkin's lymphoma

(Rappaport)	(NLI)
Nodular	
Lymphocytic poorly differentiated	Small follicle centre cell (FCC)
Mixed lymphocytic/histiocytic	Mixed small and large FCC
'Histiocytic'	Large FCC
Diffuse	
Lymphocytic well differentiated	Lymphocytic well differentiated
	Lymphocytic intermediate
Lymphocytic poorly differentiated	Lymphocytic poorly differentiated
Mixed lymphocytic/histiocytic	Mixed small lymphoid and large undifferentiated cell
'Histiocytic'	Undifferentiated large cell

3. Burkitt's lymphoma

C. **Other malignancies**
   1. Secondary tumours
   2. Leukaemias
   3. Myeloma
   4. Lymphoplasmacytoid tumour
   5. Immunoblastic sarcoma
   6. Malignant histiocytosis (histiocytic medullary reticulosis)

THYMUS
   1. Congenital disorders
      (i)   Aplasia
      (ii) Hypoplasia
   associated with defects in cellular immunity (*see* p. 47)
   2. Hyperplasia
   3. Thymoma
      Varieties
      (i)   Lymphocytic
      (ii) Lymphoepithelial
      (iii) Epithelial
      (iv) Spindle cell
      Associations with thymoma
      (i)   Myasthenia gravis
      (ii) Red cell aplasia

(iii)   Agammaglobulinaemia
(iv)   Thrombocytopenia
(v)   Cushing's syndrome
(vi)   Auto-immune conditions, especially S.L.E.
(vii) Dermatomyositis and polymyositis
(vii) Myocarditis

FURTHER READING

Harrison, C.V. (1975) Lymph-node diseases. In *Recent Advances in Pathology,* 9, ed. Harrison, C.V. & Weinbren, K., p. 73. Edinburgh: Churchill Livingstone.
Rosai, J. & Levine, G.D. (1976) Tumors of the thymus. *Atlas of Tumor Pathology,* 2nd series, 13. Montvale, N.J.: A.F.I.P.S. Press.

Endocrine system

ADRENAL CORTEX
A. Reactions to stress
1. Lipid depletion (compact-cell change)
   - (i) Focal
   - (ii) Diffuse
2. Degenerative changes in the zona fasciculata cells
3. Haemorrhage

B. Hypercorticalism results in three main syndromes
1. Cushing's syndrome
   Primary
   - (i) Cortical hyperplasia
     - a. Diffuse
     - b. Nodular
   - (ii) Adenoma
   - (iii) Carcinoma
   Secondary
   - (i) ACTH and corticosteroid administration
   - (ii) Pituitary adenoma (basophil or chromophobe)
   - (iii) Non-endocrine tumours producing ACTH
     - a. Carcinoma of the bronchus (oat-cell type)
     - b. Thymoma
     - c. Medullary carcinoma of thyroid
     - d. Islet cell tumours of pancreas
   Effects
   - (i) Obesity
   - (ii) Hypertension
   - (iii) Osteoporosis
   - (iv) Hyperglycaemia
   - (v) Myopathy
   - (vi) Atrophic change in skin
   - (vii) Polycythaemia
   - (viii) Pituitary changes—Crooke's hyaline degeneration in basophils
   - (ix) Susceptibility to infection
2. Conn's syndrome
   Primary aldosteronism due to
   - (i) Cortical adenoma
   - (ii) Diffuse or nodular hyperplasia
   - (iii) Carcinoma
   Effects
   - (i) Hypertension
   - (ii) Muscle weakness (hypokalaemia)
   - (iii) Polyuria and polydipsia
   - (iv) Hypernatraemia

3. Adreno-genital syndrome
   Causes
   (i) Congenital adrenal hyperplasia resulting from a specific enzyme deficiency (see p. 104)
   (ii) Cortical adenoma) in older children
   (iii) Carcinoma   ) and in adults
   Effects
   (i) Congenital type
       a. Male—enlargement of the penis, rapid growth, early fusion of epiphyses
       b. Female—pseudohermaphrodite, hirsutism, rapid growth
   In addition both may develop hypertension and salt-losing crises
   (ii) Adults
       a. Female—amenorrhoea, hirsutism, atrophy of the breasts, enlarged clitoris, male musculature
       b. Male—no clinical effects

C. Hypocorticalism

1. Acute adrenal insufficiency resulting from
   (i) Haemorrhagic necrosis
       a. Shock and stress reactions
       b. Septicaemia (Waterhouse-Friderichsen syndrome)
       c. Neonatal hypoxia/birth injury
   (ii) Sudden deterioration of chronic insufficiency of the adrenal cortex
2. Chronic adrenal insufficiency resulting from:
   (i) Pituitary/hypothalamic disorders
       a. Simmond's disease
       b. Sheehan's syndrome
       c. Iatrogenic
   (ii) Adrenal diseases
       a. Atrophy (idiopathic)
       b. Tuberculosis
       c. Amyloidosis
       d. Fungal infections—histoplasmosis, torulosis, coccidioidomycosis, blastomycosis,
       e. Metastatic carcinoma
       f. Haemochromatosis
       g. Following haemorrhagic necrosis
       h. Congenital disorders—hypoplasia with cytomegaly, adreno-genital syndrome
   (iii) Suppression of ACTH production by treatment with corticosteroids

Effects
a. Increased skin pigmentation
b. Hypotension
c. Muscle weakness
d. Hypoglycaemia
e. Normochromic anaemia
f. Hyponatraemia
g. Hyperkalaemia
h. Reduced renal excretion of water, ammonium and urea

ADRENAL MEDULLA

1. Phaeochromocytoma
A tumour of the catecholamine-producing chromaffin cells resulting in paroxysmal hypertension.
Associations
(i) Familial disease—autosomal dominant inheritance
(ii) Neurofibromatosis
(iii) von Hippel-Lindau disease
(iv) Medullary carcinoma of thyroid
(v) Parathyroid adenomas
Sites
(i) Adrenal medulla
(ii) Ectopic—mostly in the organs of Zuckerkandl around the origin of the inferior mesenteric artery
(iii) Multiple
Behaviour
Most are benign, about 10% are malignant.
Metastases are found in lymph glands, lungs, liver and bone

2. Neuroblastoma
A highly malignant tumour of neuroblasts, cells which normally mature into sympathetic ganglion cells. It is a common tumour of childhood.
Sites
(i) Adrenal medulla
(ii) Sympathetic chain in posterior mediastinum and abdomen
(iii) Rare sites, e.g. jaw, bladder
Spread
(i) Direct local infiltration
(ii) Lymph glands
(iii) Blood spread
a. Skeletal metastases especially to skull and orbit (Hutchinson type)
b. Multiple deposits in the liver (Pepper type)

3. Ganglioneuroma
'Mature' form of neuroblastic tumour with plentiful ganglion cells. These have a much better prognosis.
Both tumours may be associated with catecholamine production.

DIABETES MELLITUS

A metabolic disorder characterised by impaired utilisation of carbohydrates and disturbances in lipid and protein metabolism resulting from an absolute or relative deficiency of insulin.

Aetiology
1. Primary (idiopathic)
   (i) Juvenile
   (ii) Maturity-onset
2. Secondary
   (i) Pancreatic causes
      a. Pancreatitis
      b. Carcinoma of the pancreas
      c. Haemochromatosis
      d. Pancreatectomy
      e. 'Glucagonoma'
   (ii) Adrenal causes
      a. Cushing's syndrome
      b. Phaeochromocytoma
   (iii) Pituitary—acromegaly
   (iv) Thyroid—thyrotoxicosis
   (v) Drugs—thiazides

Pathological features
1. Islets of Langerhans
   (i) Degranulation of ß-cells
   (ii) Hyaline deposits and amyloidosis
   (iii) Fibrosis
   (iv) Hydropic degeneration of ß-cells
   (v) Lymphocytic infiltration
2. Kidney
   (i) Arteries and arterioles
      a. Atherosclerosis
      b. Arteriolosclerosis—afferent and efferent
   (ii) Glomeruli
      a. Diffuse glomerulosclerosis
      b. Nodular glomerulosclerosis (Kimmelstiel-Wilson lesion)
      c. Exudative lesions—fibrin cap, capsular drops
   (iii) Tubules
      a. Glycogen accumulation (Armanni-Ebstein lesion)
      b. Fatty change
   (iv) Interstitium
      a. Acute or chronic pyelonephritis
      b. Fibrosis
      c. Necrotising papillitis
3. Cardiovascular lesions
   (i) Arteries
      a. Atherosclerosis—gangrene, myocardial infarction
      b. Monckeberg's sclerosis (more common in diabetics)
   (ii) Arteriolosclerosis
   (iii) Microangiopathy

4. Ocular lesions
   (i) Capillary microaneurysms
   (ii) Retinitis proliferans resulting from repeated haemorrhages
   (iii) Thrombosis of the central retinal vein
   (iv) Cataracts
5. Liver
   (i) Fatty change
   (ii) Glycogenic vacuolation of hepatocyte nuclei
6. Gall-bladder
   (i) Cholesterolosis ⎫ incidence increased
   (ii) Gall-stones ⎭
7. Neurological lesions
   (i) Atherosclerotic neuropathy
   (ii) Diabetic pseudotabes
   (iii) Motor neuropathy
   (iv) Autonomic neuropathy
       a. Impotence
       b. Diarrhoea
       c. Atonic stomach
       d. Disturbed oesophageal peristalsis
       e. Bladder disfunction
8. Skin
   (i) Xanthomata
   (ii) Necrobiosis lipoidica diabeticorum
   (iii) Infections
       a. Pyogenic—boils, carbuncles
       b. Fungal
9. Lungs
   Increased risk of infection
       a. Bronchopneumonia
       b. Tuberculosis

PITUITARY

1. Pituitary insufficiency
   Aetiology
   (i) Ischaemic necrosis, especially post-partum (Sheehan's syndrome)
   (ii) Tumours
       a. Chromophobe adenoma
       b. Craniopharyngioma
       c. Cholesteatoma
       d. Metastatic
   (iii) Granulomata
       a. Sarcoidosis
       b. Tuberculosis
       c. Congenital syphilis
       d. Idiopathic giant-cell type
   (iv) Infiltrations
       a. Amyloidosis
       b. Hand-Schüller-Christian disease
   (v) Trauma

Anterior pituitary
Results
  (i)   Simmond's disease
      a. Loss of pigment
      b. Loss of hair
      c. Mental deterioration
      d. Genital atrophy
      e. Myxoedema
  (ii) Frohlich's syndrome—adipose-genital dystrophy
  (iii) Lorain-type dwarfism
Posterior pituitary
Results
  (i)   Diabetes insipidus
2. Pituitary hyperfunction
  (i)   Acidophil adenoma
      a. Gigantism
      b. Acromegaly
  (ii) Basophil adenoma
      a. Cushing's syndrome

THYROID

A. Congenital disorders
1. Aplasia
2. Hypoplasia
3. Thyroglossal duct/cyst/fistula
4. Lingual thyroid

B. Thyroiditis
1. Infection
  (i)   Acute non-specific
  (ii) Tuberculosis
  (iii) Sarcoidosis
  (iv) Actinomycosis
2. Immune mechanisms
  (i)   Hashimoto's disease
  (ii) Focal lymphocytic thyroiditis
3. Physical agents
  (i)   Irradiation
  (ii) Trauma
4. Unknown aetiology
  (i)   Sub-acute (giant-cell) thyroiditis—de Quervain's disease
  (ii) Fibrous thyroiditis (Riedel's struma)

C. Hyperthyroidism
Aetiology. The usual cause is:
1. Diffuse thyroid hyperplasia
but may result from:
2. Overactivity of a multinodular goitre
3. Functional (toxic) adenoma
4. Hashimoto's disease (rarely)

Diffuse thyroid hyperplasia (Graves' disease)
Aetiology
- (i)   ? Long-acting thyroid stimulator—an immunoglobulin
- (ii) ? Pituitary hyperfunction with excess TSH production

Organ changes
- (i) Thyroid
  - a. Enlargement
  - b. Columnar epithelial cells
  - c. Papillary proliferations of epithelium
  - d. Diminished colloid
  - e. Focal lymphocytic infiltration
- (ii) Exophthalmos
  - a. Oedema of the orbital contents
  - b. Increase in adipose tissue in orbits
  - c. Degeneration and fibrosis in extra-ocular muscles
- (iii) Pre-tibial myxoedema
- (iv) Lymphoid hyperplasia
- (v) Heart
  - a. Left ventricular hypertrophy
  - b. Focal myocardial necrosis
- (vi) Adrenal—hyperplasia
- (vii) Skeletal muscle
  - a. Atrophy
  - b. Adipose infiltration
  - c. Vacuolisation
- (viii) Bones
  - a. Osteoporosis
  - b. 'Thyroid acropathy'—finger-clubbing resulting from sub-periosteal new bone formation

D. Multinodular goitre
Aetiology
1. Iodine deficiency
2. Drug-induced (goitrogens)
   - (i) Iodides
   - (ii) Thioureas
   - (iii) PAS, etc.
3. Inborn errors of metabolism (dyshormonogenic goitre)
   - (i) Defective iodide trapping
   - (ii) Failure to oxidise iodide to iodine prior to incorporation into tyrosine
   - (iii) Failure to couple mono-and diiodotyrosine to form T_3 and T_4
   - (iv) Failure to de-iodinate iodine containing by-products of T_3/T_4 synthesis resulting from a lack of iodotyrosine dehalogenase
   - (v) An abnormal iodoprotein is produced instead of synthesis of thyroid hormones

Effects
Overactivity in some cases, hypofunction in others.
Most are euthyroid
Pressure on the trachea and oesophagus
Haemorrhage into a nodule
Malignant change

E. Hypothyroidism
1. Cretinism
   Aetiology
   (i) Aplasia
   (ii) Hypoplasia
   (iii) Inborn error of hormone synthesis
2. Myxoedema
   Aetiology
   (i) Primary
      a. Hashimoto's disease
      b. Other forms of thyroiditis
      c. Senile atrophy
      d. Iodine deficiency
      e. Goitrogenic drugs
      f. Thyroidectomy
      g. Irradiation
   (ii) Secondary
      a. Pituitary insufficiency (low TSH)

Organ changes
1. Cardiovascular system
   (i) Congestive cardiomyopathy
      a. Increased mucopolysaccharide in the interstitium
      b. Mucoid vacuolation of myocardial fibres
   (ii) Atherosclerosis resulting from hypercholesterolaemia
2. Myxoedema
   Infiltration of the skin and other tissues by mucoid oedema
3. Central nervous system
   (i) Mental deterioration
   (ii) Pyschosis
   (iii) Stupor and coma

F. Tumours
1. Benign
   (i) Follicular adenoma

   Variants
      a. Colloid adenoma
      b. Fetal adenoma
      c. Hürthle cell adenoma
   (ii) Teratoma (very rare)
2. Malignant
   (i) Well-differentiated carcinoma
      a. Follicular
      b. Papillary
      c. Mixed pattern

(ii) Undifferentiated carcinoma
    a. Anaplastic
    b. Medullary carcinoma (with amyloid in stroma)
(iii) Rare tumours
    a. Squamous carcinoma (by metaplasia)
    b. Sarcoma
    c. Lymphoma

PARATHYROID

A. Congenital
1. Abnormal number 2 – 5
2. Abnormal position, e.g. mediastinum

B. Hyperparathyroidism
Aetiology (see p. 113)
Effects
1. Bone
    (i) Osteitis fibrosa cystica
    (ii) Giant-cell granulomas ('brown tumours')
2. Metastatic calcification in
    (i) Kidneys
        a. Nephrocalcinosis
        b. Renal calculi
    (ii) Blood vessels
    (iii) Lung
    (iv) Stomach
3. Peptic ulceration
4. Chronic pancreatitis

C. Hypoparathyroidism
Aetiology
1. Surgical removal in thyroidectomy
2. 'Idiopathic'
    (i) Hypoplasia/aplasia (as in Di George's syndrome)
    (ii) Atrophy (? auto-immune)
3. Pseudo-hypoparathyroidism (Albright)
Effects
1. Tetany
2. Mental disturbances
3. Epilepsy
4. Papilloedema
5. Ectodermal changes
    (i) Dry skin/brittle nails
    (ii) Eczema
    (iii) Moniliasis
6. Cataracts
7. Calcification of the basal ganglia

FURTHER READING

Doniach, I. (1977) Histopathology of the anterior pituitary. *Clinics in Endocrinology and Metabolism,* 6, No. 1, 21.

Hedinger, C. & Sobin, L.H. (1974) Histological typing of thyroid tumours. *International Histological Classification of Tumours,* 11. Geneva: W.H.O.

Kay, S. (1976) Hyperplasia and neoplasia of the adrenal gland. *Pathology Annual,* 11, 103. New York: Appleton Century Crofts.

Kay, S. (1976) The abnormal parathyroid. *Human Pathology,* 7, 127.

Symington, T. (1969) *Functional Pathology of the Human Adrenal Gland.* Edinburgh: E. & S. Livingstone.

Musculoskeletal system

SKELETAL MUSCLE
A. Muscular dystrophy
1. Myotonic
   (i) Myotonia dystrophica
   (ii) Congenital myotonia (Thomsen's disease)
   (iii) Paramyotonia congenita
2. Non-myotonic
   (i) Duchenne type (pseudo-hypertrophic)
   (ii) Becker type
   (iii) Facioscapulohumeral
   (iv) Limb-girdle
   (v) Distal muscular type
   (vi) Ocular muscular type

B. Myopathies
1. Congenital
   (i) Benign congenital hypotonia
   (ii) Fibre type disproportion
   (iii) Central core disease
   (iv) Nemaline myopathy
   (v) Myotubular myopathy
   (vi) Arthrogryphosis multiplex congenita
2. Metabolic
   (i) Glycogenoses
      a. Type V (McArdle's)
      b. Type VIII
   (ii) Periodic paralysis syndromes
      a. Hypokalaemic
      b. Hyperkalaemic
      c. Normokalaemic
   (iii) Hypercalcaemia
3. Endocrine
   (i) Hyperthyroidism
   (ii) Hypothyroidism
   (iii) Hyperparathyroidism (unrelated to plasma calcium)
   (iv) Cushing's syndrome
   (v) Hyperaldosteronism
   (vi) Hypopituitarism
4. Toxic
   (i) Steroids
   (ii) Chloroquine
   (iii) Alcohol
   (iv) ? Malignant hyperpyrexia after general anaesthesia

5. Collagen diseases
   (i)   Acute rheumatic fever
   (ii) SLE
   (iii) Polyarteritis nodosa
   (iv) Polymyalgia rheumatica
6. Infection/infestation
   (i)   Coxsackie B virus (Bornholm)
   (ii) Syphilis
   (iii) Toxoplasmosis
   (iv) Trypanosomiasis
   (v)   Trichinosis
   (vi) Cysticercosis
7. Carcinoma-associated
   (i)   Neuromyopathy
   (ii) Myopathy
   (iii) Myasthenic-myopathic syndrome
8. Sarcoidosis

C. Myasthenia gravis

D. Tumours
1. Granular cell myoblastoma
2. Rhabdomyosarcoma
   (i)   Embryonal alveolar type
   (ii) Embryonal botryoid type
   (iii) Adult pleomorphic type

FIBROMATOSES
A. Congenital and juvenile
1. Fibrous hamartoma of infancy
2. Fibromatosis colli (congenital torticollis)
3. Infantile fibromatosis
   (i)   Dermal
   (ii) Diffuse
4. Juvenile fibromatosis
5. Juvenile aponeurotic fibroma
6. Congenital generalised fibromatosis

B. Miscellaneous types
1. Palmar fibromatosis (Dupuytren's contracture) and its plantar
   variant
2. Musculo-aponeurotic fibromatosis (desmoids)
3. Mesenteric fibromatosis
4. Hereditary gingival fibromatosis
5. Generalised multifocal fibromatosis

BONES
A. Congenital
1. Achondroplasia
2. Dyschondroplasia
3. Chondro-osteodystrophy (Morquio)
4. Osteogenesis imperfecta
5. Osteopetrosis
6. Marfan's syndrome
7. Gargoylism (Hunter-Hurler)

B. Inflammatory
1. Non-specific suppurative osteomyelitis
   Features
   (i)   Pus formation
   (ii) Necrosis of bone resulting from toxic and ischaemic injury (sequestrum)
   (iii) Reactive new bone formation (involucrum)
   (iv) Drainage of pus via cloacae and sinuses to the skin
   Complications
   (i)   Septicaemia
   (ii) Metastatic abscesses
   (iii) Suppurative arthritis
   (iv) Amyloidosis
2. Tuberculosis
3. Syphilis
   (i)   Osteochondritis
   (ii) Periosteitis with cortical thickening—sabre thickening
   (iii) Gummatous destruction—'worm eaten' skull

C. Osteoporosis
Reduction in calcified bone mass—generalised atrophy of bone. The disease probably represents an involutional or ageing phenomenon in which there is diminished osteoblastic activity without a corresponding reduction in osteoclasis.
   Aetiology
1. Idiopathic
   (i)   Senile
   (ii) Postmenopausal
2. Malnutrition
3. Hypovitaminosis C
4. Prolonged immobilisation
5. Endocrine
   (i)   Corticosteroid treatment/Cushing's syndrome
   (ii) Hyperthyroidism
   (iii) Acromegaly
   (iv) Hypopituitarism
6. Chronic liver and renal disease

D. Osteomalacia/rickets

Inadequate mineralisation of bone matrix resulting in a relative increase in the amount of osteoid.

Aetiology
1. Vitamin D deficiency
    (i) Malabsorption syndromes
    (ii) Dietary deficiency
    (iii) No exposure to sunlight
2. Associated with hypophosphataemia
    (i) Renal tubular acidosis
    (ii) Familial hypophosphataemia (vitamin-D resistant)
    (iii) Fanconi's syndrome
    (iv) Part of renal osteodystrophy
3. Defective mineralisation but with normal calcium, phosphorus and vitamin D levels
    (i) Hypophosphatasia
    (ii) Fluoride excess

E. Paget's disease (Osteitis deformans)

A combination of osteoclastic resorption of normal bone and osteoblastic regeneration of primitive coarse-fibred bone lying in a richly-vascular fibrous stroma.

Types
1. Monostotic—e.g. tibia
2. Polyostotic—pelvis, skull, femur, tibia
3. Localised—sharply outlined resorptive area in the skull (osteoporosis circumscripta)

Complications
1. Deformity
2. Pathological fracture
3. Encroachment on foramina producing nerve defects
4. Flattening of the base of the skull (platybasia)
5. Cardiac failure—high output required because of vascular shunts
6. Development of sarcoma (1 – 2%)
7. Hypercalcaemia when immobilised

F. Tumours

Osteogenic tumours
  Benign
1. Osteoma
2. Osteoid osteoma
3. Osteoblastoma—'giant osteoid osteoma'
  Malignant
1. Osteogenic sarcoma
2. Parosteal osteosarcoma

Cartilagenous tumours
  Benign
  1. Osteochondroma—osteocartilaginous exostosis
      (i)   Single
      (ii) Multiple
  2. Chondroma
      (i)   Eccondroma
      (ii) Enchondroma
            Multiple in Ollier's disease
            Associated with haemangiomata in Maffucci's syndrome
  3. Chondroblastoma—Codman's tumour
  4. Chondromyxoid fibroma
  Malignant
  1. Chondrosarcoma
  2. Mesenchymal chondrosarcoma

Fibrous tumours
  Benign
  1. Non-osteogenic fibroma
  2. Ossifying fibroma
  3. Fibromyxoma
  Malignant
      Fibrosarcoma

Giant-cell 'tumours'
  1. True giant-cell tumour
  2. Giant-cell reparative granuloma of jaw
  3. 'Brown tumours' of hyperparathyroidism
  4. Simple bone cyst
  5. Aneurysmal bone cyst

Tumours arising from bone-marrow
  1. Leukaemias
  2. Multiple myeloma
  3. Reticulum cell sarcoma

Other tumours
  1. Ewing's tumour
  2. Chordoma
  3. Haemangioma
  4. Neurofibroma
  5. Eosinophil granuloma
  6. Adamantinoma of long bones

Metastatic tumours
Childhood—neuroblastoma
Adult—
1. Osteosclerotic carcinomas
   (i) Prostate
   (ii) Breast
   (iii) Adenocarcinoma of bronchus
   (iv) Signet-ring type of gastric carcinoma
2. Osteolytic carcinomas
   (i) Renal
   (ii) Thyroid
   (iii) Colon
   (iv) Breast
3. Unchanged—oat-cell carcinoma of bronchus

OSTEOARTHROSIS
Aetiology
1. Primary—degeneration
2. Secondary
   (i) Trauma
   (ii) Obesity
   (iii) Osteochondritis
   (iv) Developmental—e.g. congenital dislocation
   (v) Haemophilia
   (vi) Ochronosis
   (vii) Acromegaly
Features
1. Fibrillation of cartilage
2. Fragmentation
3. Exposure of bone with thickening—eburnation
4. Marginal new bone formation—osteophytes
5. Fibrosis of underlying bone—radiological 'cysts'

RHEUMATOID ARTHRITIS
Features
1. Synovial inflammation
2. Accumulation of fibrinoid material on the synovium
3. Enlargement of synovial villi resulting from oedema, proliferation and cellular infiltration (lymphocytes and plasma-cells)
4. Erosion of cartilage at the margins
5. Replacement by granulation tissue—pannus
6. Fusion of articular surfaces by fibrosis—ankylosis, or subluxation of the joint

Extra-articular lesions of rheumatoid disease
1. Nodules
    (i)   Subcutaneous tissue
    (ii)   Lung and pleura
    (iii) Heart—base of valves
    (iv)   Dura mater
2. Bones
    (i)   Periarthrodal osteoporosis
    (ii)   Generalised osteoporosis resulting from
           a. immobilisation
           b. steroid therapy
3. Heart
    (i)   Nodules
    (ii)   Pericarditis
    (iii) Coronary arteritis
4. Blood vessels
    (i)   vasculitis
    (ii)   intimal proliferation leading to occlusion
5. Lungs
    (i)   Diffuse interstitial fibrosis
    (ii)   Nodular lung disease
    (iii) Rheumatoid pneumoconiosis (Caplan's syndrome)
6. Lymph glands—follicular hyperplasia
7. Secondary amyloidosis
8. Kidneys—secondary involvement due to
    (i)   Arteritis
    (ii)   Amyloid
    (iii) Analgesics
9. Eyes
    (i)   Keratoconjunctivitis sicca
    (ii)   Episcleritis
    (iii) Scleromalacia perforans
    (iv)   Uveitis
10. Nerves
    (i)   Secondary to vasculitis
    (ii)   Compression
    (iii) Amyloidosis
    (iv)   Drugs
11. Muscle
    (i)   Atrophy secondary to neuropathy
    (ii)   Steroid myopathy
12. Thyroid
    Increased incidence of
    (i)   Thyrotoxicosis
    (ii)   Hashimoto's disease
13. Sjögren's syndrome

FURTHER READING

Bethlem, J. (1970) *Muscle Pathology; Introduction and Atlas.* London: North-Holland.

Duchen, L.W. (1975) Pathology of the innervation of skeletal muscle. *In Recent Advances in Pathology,* 9, ed. Harrison, C.V. & Weinbren, K. p. 217. Edinburgh: Churchill Livingstone.

Jaffe, H.L. (1958) *Tumors and Tumorous Conditions of the Bones and Joints.* Philadelphia: Lea & Febiger.

Jaffe, H.L. (1972) *Metabolic, Degenerative and Inflammatory Diseases of Bones and Joints.* Philadelphia: Lea and Febiger.

Mackenzie, D.H. (1970) *Differential Diagnosis of Fibroblastic Disorders.* Oxford: Blackwell.

Mackenzie, D.H. (1975) Miscellaneous soft-tissue sarcomas. In *Recent Advances in Pathology,* 9, ed. Harrison, C.V. & Weinbren, K. p. 183. Edinburgh: Churchill Livingstone.

Stout, A.P. & Lattes, R. (1967) Tumors of the soft tissues. *Atlas of Tumor Pathology,* 2nd series, 1. Montvale, N.J.: A.F.I.P.S. Press.

Auto-immune diseases

SYSTEMIC LUPUS ERYTHEMATOSUS
Aetiology
Auto-immune reactions initiated by
1. Genetic predisposition
2. Drugs
   (i) Hydralazine
   (ii) Procainamide
   (iii) Penicillin
   (iv) α-Methyl dopa
3. Viruses
4. Sunlight
Features
1. Skin
   (i) Liquefaction/degeneration at the dermal-epidermal junction
   (ii) Homogenisation of collagen fibres
   (iii) Fibrinoid necrosis in blood vessels
   (distinguish from discoid LE)
2. Kidneys
   (i) Diffuse proliferative GN (immune complex type)
   (ii) Focal GN
   (iii) Membranous GN—'wire loop' lesions
   (iv) Vasculitis
3. Heart
   (i) Pericarditis
   (ii) Myocarditis
   (iii) Endocarditis—atypical verrucous endocarditis (Libman-Sacks)
4. Lungs and pleura
   (i) Pleurisy
   (ii) Pneumonitis
   (iii) Arteritis
5. Joints—inflammation, but not destruction as in R.A.
6. Spleen
   (i) Perisplenitis
   (ii) 'Onion-skin' arteriolar thickening
7. Lymph glands
   (i) Follicular hyperplasia
   (ii) Focal necrosis
8. CNS
   (i) Epilepsy
   (ii) Mental/hypothalamic features
   (iii) Myasthenic syndrome

PROGRESSIVE SYSTEMIC SCLEROSIS
Features
1. Skin
   (i) Pigmentation
   (ii) Epidermal atrophy with loss of appendages
   (iii) Dermal oedema and separation of collagen
   (iv) Calcinosis
2. Lungs
   (i) Interstitial fibrosis—honeycomb lung
   (ii) Vascular changes
3. Kidneys
   (i) Basement membrane thickening
   (ii) Fibrinoid necrosis in arterioles
   (iii) Cortical infarcts
4. Alimentary tract
   (i) Collagenous thickening—hypomotility
   (ii) Villous atrophy
5. Blood vessels
   (i) Intimal proliferation and medial hypertrophy
   (ii) Fibrinoid necrosis
6. Muscle
   (i) Atrophy
   (ii) Myositis
7. Joints
   (i) Synovitis
   (ii) Synovial sclerosis
8. Heart
   (i) Myocardial fibrosis
   (ii) Pericarditis
9. Thymus
   (i) Lympho-epithelial proliferation
   (ii) Enlarged Hassall's corpuscles

POLYARTERITIS NODOSA
Disseminated necrotising inflammation affecting medium-sized and small arteries.

Features
1. Medial fibrinoid necrosis
2. Polymorph infiltration
3. Destruction of the internal elastic lamina
4. Super-imposed thrombosis
5. Fibroblastic proliferation
6. Infiltration by lymphocytes, plasma cells, eosinophils
7. Increasing collagenisation
Results
1. Haemorrhage
2. Infarction
3. Aneurysmal dilatation

Organs affected
1. Kidneys
    (i)   Focal necrosis
    (ii) Proliferation—crescent formation
    (iii) Granular deposits and fibrin (GBM)
2. Heart
3. Liver
4. G.I. tract
5. Lungs
6. Peripheral nerves

FURTHER READING

Burnet, Sir F.M. (1972) *Auto-immunity and Auto-immune Disease*. Lancaster: Medical and Technical Publishing.

Gardner, D.L. (1965) *Pathology of the Connective Tissue Diseases*. London: Arnold.

Holt, P.J.L. (Ed.) (1975) *Current Topics in Connective Tissue Disease*. Edinburgh: Churchill Livingstone.

Nervous system

BRAIN AND SPINAL CORD

A. Congenital
1. Abnormalities of fusion
   - (i) Spina bifida occulta
   - (ii) Meningocoele
   - (iii) Meningomyelocoele
   - (iv) Myelocoele-rachiscisis
   - (v) Encephalocoele
   - (vi) Anencephaly—cranioscisis
2. Abnormalities of cleavage
   - (i) Cyclopia
   - (ii) Arrhinencephaly
   - (iii) Telencephalon impar
3. Abnormalities of migration of neuroblasts
   - (i) Ectopias
   - (ii) Pachygyria
   - (iii) Microgyria

B. Hydrocephalus
1. Obstruction to CSF flow
   - (i) Congenital malformations
     - a. Arnold-Chiari malformation
     - b. Stenosis of the aqueduct
     - c. Dandy-Walker syndrome
     - d. Atresia or stenosis of the foramina of Magendie and Luschka
   - (ii) Post-inflammatory
     - a. Meningitis
     - b. Trauma
   - (iii) Space-occupying lesions
     - a. Neoplasms
     - b. Cysts
     - c. Abscesses
     - d. Haematomata
2. Defective absorption
   - (i) Adhesions over the cerebral hemispheres
   - (ii) Organised exudate around arachnoidal villi
   - (iii) Thrombosis of the major venous sinuses
3. Excessive production of CSF.
   Papilloma of the choroid plexus (very rare)
4. Mechanism unknown
   - (i) Idiopathic cases
   - (ii) 'Normal pressure hydrocephalus'

C. Meningitis

Predisposing factors
1. Local infection, e.g. otitis media, mastoiditis
2. Distant infection, e.g. tuberculosis, pneumococcal pneumonia
3. Trauma, e.g. frontal fractures

Varieties
1. Pyogenic (purulent or suppurative)
   (i) Neonatal
       a. Gram-negative bacilli:
          E. coli
          B. proteus
          Pseudomonas spp
       b. Streptococcus
       c. Staphylococcus
       d. *Haemophilus influenzae*
       e. *Listeria monocytogenes*
   (ii) Infant
       a. *H. influenzae*
       b. Meningococcus
       c. Pneumococcus, etc.
   (iii) Children and young adults
       a. Meningococcus
       b. Pneumococcus, etc.
   (iv) Elderly
       a. Pneumococcus, etc.
2. 'Aseptic'
   (i) Viruses
       a. Mumps
       b. Enteroviruses:
          ECHO
          Coxsackie
          Poliomyelitis
       c. Herpes zoster
       d. EB virus
       e. Lymphocytic choriomeningitis virus
   (ii) Tuberculosis
   (iii) Syphilis
   (iv) Sarcoidosis
   (v) Fungi
       a. Histoplasmosis
       b. Coccidioidomycosis
       c. Mucormycosis
       d. Torulosis
   (vi) Rickettsia
   (vii) Protozoa
       a. Toxoplasmosis
       b. Free-living amoebae:
          Hartmanella
          Naegleria

D. Cerebral abscess
Predisposing factors
1. Local infection, e.g.
   - (i) Otitis media/mastoiditis
   - (ii) Sinusitis
   - (iii) Venous sinus phlebitis
2. Distant infection with blood spread, e.g.
   - (i) Bronchiectasis
   - (ii) Empyema
   - (iii) Lung abscess
   - (iv) Acute endocarditis
3. Penetrating injury or surgery
4. Cyanotic heart disease, organisms by-pass the pulmonary vascular 'filter'

E. Viral encephalitis
1. Primary—arboviruses
   - (i) Transmitted by mosquitos:
     Group A—Eastern equine encephalitis; Western equine encephalitis; Venezuelan equine encephalitis
     Group B—St. Louis encephalitis; Murray Valley encephalitis; Japanese encephalitis
   - (ii) Tick-borne encephalitis:
     Russian spring-summer
     Central European
     Louping ill
2. Secondary to systemic infection (which may be inapparent)
   - (i) Herpesvirus hominis
   - (ii) Mumps
   - (iii) Varicella
   - (iv) Measles
   - (v) ECHO viruses
3. Slow-virus infections
   - (i) Kuru
   - (ii) Jakob-Creutzfeldt's disease

F. Vascular disorders
1. Meningeal haemorrhage
   - (i) Extradural—haemorrhage between the skull and the dura resulting from trauma
   - (ii) Subdural—haemorrhage between the dura and the arachnoid, usually a result of trauma but may occasionally follow rupture of a berry aneurysm
   - (iii) Subarachnoid—haemorrhage between the arachnoid and pia resulting from:
     a. Rupture of a 'berry' aneurysm
     b. Extension from an intracerebral haemorrhage
     c. Traumatic

2. Intracerebral haemorrhage
    (i)   Massive haemorrhage resulting from
          a. Hypertensive cerebral vascular disease
          b. Ruptured aneurysm
          c. Trauma
          d. Bleeding diathesis
          e. Angiomas/vascular malformations
          f. Bleeding into a tumour
    (ii) Scattered punctate haemorrhages
          a. Cerebral contusion
          b. Asphyxia
          c. Fat or air embolism
          d. Infections—viral encephalitis, septicaemia
          e. Bleeding diathesis
3. Anoxic—ischaemic injury
    Aetiology
    (i)   Cardiac arrest
    (ii) Systemic hypotension
    (iii) Respiratory failure
    (iv) Severe anaemia
    (v)   Poisoning—carbon monoxide, nitrous oxide etc
    (vi) High altitude
    Regions most vulnerable to hypoxia
    (i)   Hippocampus
    (ii) Purkinje cells of the cerebellum
    (iii) Small pyramidal cells of frontal and occipital cortex
    (iv) Amygdaloid nucleus
    (v)   Brain-stem
    Cellular changes
    (i)   Neuronal degeneration and disappearance
          a. Swelling and pallor of cytoplasm
          b. Loss of Nissl substance
          c. Nuclear swelling
          d. Pyknosis and acidophilic shrinkage necrosis
          e. Karyolysis
          f. Neuronophagia
    (ii) Astrocytic proliferation and glial scarring
4. Non-infarctive ischaemia
    resulting from gradual narrowing of small arteries and
    arterioles by
    (i)   Hyaline thickening of the media (Hypertension/Diabetes)
    (ii) Adventitial sclerosis
    Effects
    (i)   Formation of lacunae—small cystic cavities 2 – 10 mm
          diameter
    (ii) Granular cortical atrophy in 'watershed' areas
    (iii) Status cribrosus—1 – 2 mm zones of degeneration
          around small perforating vessels of the basal ganglia
    (iv) Binswanger's subcortical encephalopathy—focal
          demyelination of white matter due to selective
          involvement of deeper arterial branches

5. Cerebral infarction
    Aetiology
    (i)   Occlusion or narrowing of cerebral, vertebral and
          internal carotid arteries by
          a. Atherosclerosis
          b. Thrombosis
          c. Embolism
    (ii) Arteritis/thrombosis
          a. Complicating meningitis
          b. Endarteritis obliterans in syphilis
    c.   Polyarteritis nodosa
          d. SLE
          e. Giant-cell arteritis
    Cellular changes
    (i)   Ischaemic degeneration of neurones
    (ii) Myelin pallor
    (iii) Destruction of myelin sheaths and axis cylinders
    (iv) Macrophage activity—ingestion of myelin and red-blood
          cells
    (v)   Astrocytic proliferation—gliosis
    Macroscopic changes
    (i)   Softening
    (ii) Liquefactive (colliquative) necrosis
    (iii) Cyst formation

G. **Disorders of myelination**
    1. Defective myelination due to an inherited defect
        (i)   Metachromatic leucodystrophy (accumulation of
              sulphatide)
        (ii) Krabbe's disease (galactocerebroside)
        (iii) Pelizaeus-Merzbacher disease
        (iv) Spongiform degeneration of the white matter—Canavan
              disease
    2. Acquired demyelination
        (i)   Multiple sclerosis
              Lesions (plaques) most commonly found in
              a. Optic nerves
              b. Around the lateral ventricles
              c. Brain stem
              d. Cerebellar peduncles
              e. Dorsal spinal cord
              Microscopic features
              a. Loss of myelin
              b. Perivascular lymphocytic infiltration
              c. Marked reactive gliosis
        (ii) Neuromyelitis optica (Devic's disease—probable variant
              of MS)
        (iii) Acute disseminated encephalomyelitis
        (iv) Diffuse cerebral sclerosis (Schilder's disease)
        (v)   Subacute sclerosing panencephalitis
        (vi) Progressive multifocal leucoencephalopathy

H. Metabolic disorders
1. Neuronal lipidoses
   - (i) Tay-Sach's disease
   - (ii) Niemann-Pick's disease
   - (iii) Gaucher's disease
   - (iv) Hunter-Hurler disease
2. Phenylpyruvic oligophrenia
3. Maple-syrup urine disease
4. Galctosaemic oligophrenia
5. Porphyric myelopathy
6. Wilson's disease
7. Hallervorden-Spatz disease (iron-containing pigment in the globus pallidus and substantia nigra)

I. Degenerative disorders
1. Alzheimer's disease
   Features
   - (i) Cerebral atrophy
   - (ii) Neuronal loss
   - (iii) Senile plaques in grey matter
   - (iv) Neurofibrillar degeneration ('tangles')
2. Parkinson's disease
   - (i) Idiopathic (paralysis agitans)
     Features
     - a. Loss of pigmented neurones from the substantia nigra, locus caeruleus, and motor nucleus of X
     - b. Rounded acidophilic inclusions in neurones—Lewy bodies
     - c. Gliosis
       some cases have
     - d. Autonomic degeneration with postural hypotension (Shy-Drager syndrome)
   - (ii) Postencephalitic
     Features
     - a. Loss of pigmented neurones from the substantia nigra and occasionally from the locus caeruleus
     - b. Neurofibrillary tangles in affected neurones
     - c. Gliosis
   - (iii) Other conditions producing lesions in striato-nigral pathways (Parkinsonism)
     - a. Cerebrovascular disease
     - b. Wilson's disease
     - c. Head injury ('punch-drunk' syndrome)
     - d. Meningovascular syphilis
     - e. Carbon-monoxide poisoning
     - f. Manganese poisoning
   - (iv) Drug-induced Parkinsonism
     - a. Reserpine
     - b. Methyldopa
     - c. Phenothiazines

3. Pick's disease
4. Huntington's chorea
5. Spinocerebellar degenerations
    (i)   Friedrich's ataxia
    (ii)   Carcinomatous cerebellar degeneration
    (iii) Alcoholic cerebellar degeneration
    (iv)   Bassen-Kornzweig syndrome
        a. Cerebellar ataxia
        b. Fat retention in surface enterocytes of jejunum
        c. Abetalipoproteinaemia
        d. Acanthocytosis (red blood cells)
6. Motor neurone disease
    (i)   Progressive muscular atrophy—lower motor neurones
    (ii)   Amyotrophic lateral sclerosis—upper and lower motor
           neurones
    (iii) Primary lateral sclerosis—upper motor neurones
    (iv)   Bulbar palsy—localised
7. Subacute combined degeneration of the cord
   Demyelination of posterior and, later, lateral columns
   associated with pernicious anaemia

J. Tumours

Neuroectodermal tumours
1. Gliomas
    (i)   Astrocytoma: Grade I – IV
           (Grade IV equivalent to glioblastoma multiforme)
           Descriptive varieties of astrocytoma
        a. Fibrillary
        b. Pilocytic
        c. Gemistocytic
    (ii)   Oligodendroglioma
    (iii) Ependymoma—
           develop from the lining of the ventricular system.
           Myxopapillary ependymoma arises from the filum
           terminale
    (iv)   Polar spongioblastoma (very rare)
2. Medulloblastoma
3. Ganglioneuroma and ganglioglioma

Mesodermal tumours
1. Meningioma
    Sites
    (i)   Parasagittal
    (ii)   Spinal cord
    (iii) Sphenoidal ridge
    (iv)   Olfactory groove
    Microscopic types
    (i)   Psammomatous
    (ii)   Meningoepithelial
    (iii) Fibroblastic
    (iv)   Angiomatous

2. Neurolemmal tumours, e.g. acoustic neuroma
3. Haemangioblastoma—sometimes part of the von Hippel-Lindau syndrome
4. Reticulum cell sarcoma—Microglioma

Tumours of developmental origin
1. Craniopharyngioma
2. Cholesteatoma and dermoid cyst
3. Chordoma

Metastatic tumours from
1. Carcinoma of bronchus, breast, kidney, colon
2. Malignant melanoma of skin
3. Chorion carcinoma of the uterus

PERIPHERAL NERVES
Mononeuropathy
Lesions of individual peripheral nerves
Aetiology
1. Penetrating injury
2. Traction
3. Compression
   (i) External, e.g. tourniquet or crutch
   (ii) Internal, e.g. carpal tunnel syndrome
4. Haemorrhage into the nerve
5. Infarction, e.g. in diabetes

Multiple mononeuropathy (mononeuritis multiplex)
Discrete lesions of several nerves arising simultaneously or in succession.
1. Diabetes
2. Leprosy
3. Sarcoidosis
4. Polyarteritis nodosa
5. Amyloidosis

Polyneuropathy
Generalised involvement
1. Dietary deficiencies
   (i) Chronic alcoholism
   (ii) Sprue
   (iii) Pellagra
   (iv) Beri-Beri
   (v) Subacute combined degeneration
2. Related to infections
   (i) Acute post-infective polyneuritis (Guillain-Barré)
   (ii) Leprosy
   (iii) Diphtheria
   (iv) Infectious mononucleosis

3. Metabolic
   (i)   Diabetes mellitus
   (ii) Uraemia
   (iii) Hepatic failure
   (iv) Acute intermittent porphyria
   (v)   Amyloidosis
   (vi) Myxoedema
4. Vascular
   (i)   Polyarteritis
   (ii) SLE
5. Toxic
   (i)   Heavy metals
   (ii) Organo-phorphorus compounds
   (iii) Drugs, isoniazid and many others
6. Carcinomatous, especially bronchial
7. Heredofamilial disorders
   (i)   Peroneal muscular atrophy (Charcot-Marie-Tooth)
   (ii) Hypertrophic interstitial polyneuritis (Dejerine-Sottas)
   (iii) Hereditary sensory radicular polyneuropathy
   (iv) Refsum's disease
         a. Polyneuritis
         b. Ichthyosis
         c. Retinopathy
         d. Deafness and anosmia

Tumours
1. Neurofibroma
   (i)   Solitary
   (ii) Multiple—von Recklinghausen's disease
2. Neurilemmoma
3. Neurofibrosarcoma
4. Malignant neurilemmoma
5. Ganglioneuroma   } autonomic nervous system
6. Ganglioneuroblastoma }
7. Neuroblastoma

FURTHER READING

Blackwood, W. & Corsellis, J.A.N. (Ed.) (1976) *Greenfield's Neuropathology,* 3rd edn. London: Arnold.
Escourolle, R. & Poirier, J. (1973) *Manual of Basic Neuropathology.* Philadelphia: Saunders.
Rubinstein, L.J. (1972) Tumors·of the central nervous system. *Atlas of Tumor Pathology,* 2nd series, 6. Montvale, N.J.: A.F.I.P.S. Press.
Russell, D.S. & Rubinstein, L.J. (1977) *Pathology of Tumours of the Nervous System,* 4th edn. London: Arnold.

General references

Ackerman, L.V. & Rosai, J. (1974) *Surgical Pathology*, 5th edn. St. Louis: Mosby.

Anderson, J.R. (Ed.) (1976) *Muir's Textbook of Pathology*, 10th edn. London: Arnold.

Anderson, W.A.D. (Ed.) (1971) *Pathology*, 6th edn. St. Louis: Mosby.

Curran, R.C. & Harnden, D.G. (Eds.) (1972) *The Pathological Basis of Medicine*. London: Heinemann.

Robbins, S.L. (1974) *Pathologic Basis of Disease*. London: Saunders.

Symmers, W. St C. (Ed.) (1976) *Systemic Pathology*, 2nd edn. Vol. 1. Edinburgh: Churchill Livingstone.

Walter, J.B. & Israel, M.S. (1974) *General Pathology*, 4th edn. Edinburgh: Churchill Livingstone.

Index

Adrenal cortex, 212
Adrenal medulla, 214
Adrenogenital syndrome, 213
Alcohol, liver injury, 165
Amino-acid metabolism, errors of, 100
Amyloid, 115
Aneurysms, 78
Appendix, 157
Arteriosclerosis, 74
Arteritis, 179
Atherosclerosis, 74
Atrophy, 120
Auto-immunity, 43

Benign tumours, 128
Bilirubin metabolism, 107
Bladder, 200
Body defences, 47
Bone, 224
Breast, 206
Bronchial asthma, 186
Bronchiectasis, 185
Bronchitis, chronic, 184

Calcification, 113
Calcospherites, 114
Calculi, 114
  urinary, 198
Carbohydrate metabolism, errors of, 99
Carcinogenesis, 135
Cardiac failure, 90
Cardiomyopathy, 175
Cell, components, 1
  death, 9
  injury, 5
Cervix, 204
Childhood, tumours of, 142
Cholelithiasis, 168
Chromosome abnormalities, 97
Cirrhosis, 166
Cloudy swelling, 6
Coeliac disease, 154
Complement, 14
Congenital heart disease, 174
Congenital malformations, 96
Congestion, 90
Conn's syndrome, 212
Crohn's disease, 153

Cushing's syndrome, 212
Cytology, exfoliative, 125

Diabetes mellitus, 215
Drugs and the liver, 163
Dysplasia, 125

Embolism, 84
Encephalitis, 235
Endocarditis, infective, 177
Endometriosis, 203
Eosinophils, 31
Epididymis, 201
Exfoliative cytology, 125
Exudate, cellular, 14
  fluid, 13
  and oedema, 88

Fat, embolism, 85
  necrosis, 10
Fatty change, 7
Fibromatoses, 223
Fracture healing, 26

Gall-bladder, 168
Gangrene, 10
Giant-cells, 31
Glomerulonephritis, 194
Glycosaminoglycans, accummulation, 102

Haematological effects of tumours, 141
Haemochromatosis, 109
Haemoglobin, 105
Haemosiderosis, 109
Hamartoma, 131
Hepatitis, viral, 162
Hormonal effects of tumours, 141
Hydrocephalus, 233
Hyperbilirubinaemia, 107
Hypercorticalism, 212
Hyperplasia, 122
  of prostate, 293
Hypersensitivity, 38
Hypertension, pulmonary, 72
  systemic 66
Hyperthyroidism, 217
Hypertrophy, 121
Hypocorticalism, 213

Hypothyroidism, 219

Immune response, 36
Immunity, 47
Immunodeficiency, 45
Immunoglobulins, 37
Inflammation, acute, 12
  chemical mediators of, 15
  chronic, 29
  general responses to, 34
Injury, reactions to, 93
Invasion, 132
Iron, abnormal storage, 109
Ischaemic heart disease, 178

Jaundice, 107

Kidney diseases, 193
Kveim test, 61

Large intestine, 157
Larynx, 183
Leprosy, 57
Leucocyte migration, 13
Leukoplakia, 147
Lipid storage diseases, 102
Lipofuscins, 112
Lymphokines, 32

Macrophage, 30
Malabsorption, 154
Mammary dysplasia, 207
Melanin, 110
Membranous nephropathy, 195
Meningitis, 234
Metaplasia, 124
Metastasis, 133
Mononuclear phagocyte system, 30
Mouth, 147
Mucopolysaccharides, accumulation,
  102
Myocarditis, 175
Myopathies, 222

Necrosis, 10
Nephrocalcinosis, 199
Neuropathies, 240
Nose, 181

Oedema, 88
Oesophagus, 148
Opportunistic infection, 50
Osteoarthrosis, 224
Osteomalacia, 225
Osteoporosis, 224
Ovary, tumours of, 206

Paget's disease, of bone, 225
  of skin, 125
Pancreas, 170
Parathyroid, 220
Parkinson's disease, 238
Peptic ulcer, 151
Pericardium, 173
Phaeochromocytoma, 214
Phagocytosis, 3, 17
Pharynx, 147
Pituitary, 216
Pneumonia, 186
Polyarteritis nodosa, 231
Polymorphs, disorders of, 18
  eosinophil, 31
  neutrophil, 17
Polyps, cervical, 205
  gastric, 152
Porphyrias, 105
Portal hypertension, 166
Progressive systemic sclerosis, 231
Prostate, 200
Pulmonary, emphysema, 189
  fibrosis, 188
  hypertension, 72
  oedema, 190
Pyelonephritis, 193

Radiation, 143
Reactive lymphadenopathy, 209
Regeneration, 23
Renal tubular disorders, 197
Repair, 22
Rheumatic fever, 176
Rheumatoid arthritis, 227
Rheumatoid disease, 228

Salivary glands, 146
Sarcoidosis, 59
Shock, 94
Skin changes in malignancy, 140
Small intestine, 153
Steroid metabolism, errors of, 104
Stomach, 150
Syphilis, 61
Systemic lupus erythematosus, 230

Teratoma, 130
Testis, 201
Thrombosis, 79
Thymus, 210
Thyroiditis, 217
Trachea, 184
Transplantation, 42
Tuberculosis, 52

Tumours, 128
  childhood, 142
  classification, 129
  haematological effects, 141
  irradiation of, 145
  neuromuscular effects, 140

Tumours cont.
  spread of, 132
Ulcerative colitis, 158
Uterus, 203

Wound healing, 23